NCLEX-PN®
250 New-Format Questions
Second Edition

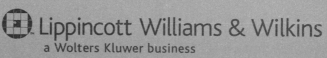

Lippincott Williams & Wilkins
a Wolters Kluwer business

Philadelphia · Baltimore · New York · London
Buenos Aires · Hong Kong · Sydney · Tokyo

STAFF

Executive Publisher
Judith A. Schilling McCann, RN, MSN

Senior Acquisitions Editor
Elizabeth Nieginski

Editorial Director
David Moreau

Clinical Director
Joan M. Robinson, RN, MSN

Senior Art Director
Arlene Putterman

Editorial Project Manager
Tracy S. Diehl

Clinical Project Manager
Carol A. Saunderson, RN, BA, BS

Editors
Karen C. Comerford, Josephine Donofrio

Clinical Editors
Tamara Kear, RN, MSN, CNN; Carol Knauff, RN, MSN, CCRN; Anita Lockhart, RNC, MSN; Anne Marie Palatnik, MSN, APN, BC; Barbara Steibling, BSN, MSN

Designers
Susan Hopkins Rodzewich (book design), Stephanie Biddle (project manager)

Digital Composition Services
Diane Paluba (manager), Joyce Rossi Biletz, Donna S. Morris

Manufacturing
Patricia K. Dorshaw (director), Beth J. Welsh

Editorial Assistants
Megan L. Aldinger, Karen J. Kirk, Linda K. Ruhf

Design Assistant
Georg W. Purvis, IV

PN2502010106—D N O S A J J M A M F J
08 07 06   10 9 8 7 6 5 4 3 2 1

Library of Congress Cataloging-in-Publication Data

NCLEX-PN 250 new-format questions : preparing for the revised NCLEX-PN.—2nd ed.
        p. ; cm.
    Includes bibliographical references and index.
    1. Practical nursing—Examinations, questions, etc. 2. Practical nursing—Outlines, syllabi, etc. 3. Practical nurses—Licenses—United States—Examinations—Study guides. I. Lippincott Williams & Wilkins. II. Title: NCLEX-PN two hundred fifty new-format questions.
    [DNLM: 1. Nursing, Practical—Examination Questions. 2. Nursing Care—Examination Questions. WY 18.2 N3368 2006]
RT55.N415 2006
610.7306'93076—dc22
ISBN 1-58255-534-6 (alk. paper)   2005029301

Contents

Contributors

Katrina Davis Allen, RN, MSN, CCRN
Nursing Faculty (ADN)
Faulkner State Community College
Bay Minette, Ala.

Kathy Cochran, RN, MSN
Director of Practical Nursing/Nursing Instructor
Coosa Valley Technical College
Rome, Ga.

Diane J. Lane, RN, MSN, BSN
HST Instructor, Vocational Nursing
Silva Health Magnet High School WPISD
El Paso, Texas

Shirley MacNeill, RN, BSN
Vocational Nursing Faculty
Lamar State College
Port Arthur, Texas

Ose G. Martinez, RN, BSN
Nursing Faculty
Central Georgia Technical College
Macon

Tracy Jo Pekar, RN, MSN, MBA
Nursing Instructor
Westmoreland County Community College
Greene County Vocational Technical School
Waynesburg, Pa.

Noel C. Piano, RN, MS
Nursing Instructor
Lafayette School of Practical Nursing
Williamsburg, Va.

Theresa Pulvano, RN, BSN
Nursing Educator
Ocean County Vocational Technical School
Toms River, N.J.

Kristi Robinia, RNC, MSN
Program Coordinator for Practical Nursing
Northern Michigan University
Marquette

Sheryl Thomas, RN, MSN
Nurse Instructor
Wayne County Community College
Detroit

You've worked hard to earn your degree. You're ready to move ahead in your career and begin your nursing practice. Only one thing stands in your way — the National Council Licensure Examination for Practical Nurses® (NCLEX-PN®).

Alternate-format questions

Every nursing student is familiar with the pressure and anxiety involved with taking the NCLEX-PN. As if the stress of the standard test questions weren't enough, however, the National Council of State Boards of Nursing (NCSBN) added five types of alternate-format questions to the NCLEX. But don't worry, *NCLEX-PN: 250 New-Format Questions,* Second Edition, is a cutting-edge review book that will help you become fully prepared for every type of question you may encounter on the NCLEX.

Multiple-response

The first type of alternate-format question is the multiple-response question. Unlike a traditional multiple-choice question, each multiple-response question has *one or more* correct answers, and it may contain more than four possible answer options. You'll recognize this type of question because you'll be asked to select *all* the answers that apply — not just the *best* answer (as may be requested in the more traditional multiple-choice questions).

When you encounter one of these questions in this review book, read the question and all possible answers carefully. Place a check mark in the box next to all options that correctly answer the question. Keep in mind that, for each multiple-response question, you must select *all correct answers* for the item to be counted as correct (one or more choices make up the correct answer). On the NCLEX, there is no partial credit in the scoring of these items.

Fill-in-the-blank

The second type of alternate-format question is the fill-in-the-blank. These questions require you to provide the answer yourself, rather than select it from a list of options. For these questions, write your answer in the blank space provided after the question. Keep in mind that these questions are based on calculation problems and require only a numerical answer. Include a decimal point if appropriate and, if necessary, perform rounding at the end of the calculation. Do not put measurements after or commas within the numerical answer.

Hot spot

The third type of alternate-format question is a question in which you will be asked to identify an area on an illustration or graphic. For these so-called "hot spot" questions, the computerized exam will ask you to place your cursor over the correct area on an illustration and click.

When reviewing such questions in this book, read the question and then mark an X on the illustration in the left-hand column to indicate your answer. In the right-hand column, correct answers are similarly indicated by an X on the duplicate illustration. Try to be as precise as possible when marking the location. As with the fill-in-the-blanks, the identification questions on the computerized exam may require extremely precise answers in order for them to be considered correct.

Drag-and-drop

The fourth type of alternate-format question is the "drag-and-drop," which requires you to use the mouse to drag and drop the answers into the correct ascending sequential order. You may also highlight the option and then click the arrow key to move the option to the answer box.

When reviewing such questions in this book, you'll see a list of unordered options followed by a series of blank answer boxes for you to fill in, in the correct order.

Chart/Exhibit

The fifth type of alternate-format question is the chart/exhibit. Although it's a multiple-choice question, this type of question requires you to base your answer on a chart or exhibit. Read the question and look at the chart or exhibit provided, and then choose from the correct answer options.

Preparing for the exam

These new alternate-format questions are sure to make the NCLEX exam even more challenging than it has been in the past. Luckily, *NCLEX-PN: 250 New-Format Questions,* Second Edition, was specifically developed to help you prepare for and excel at each of these types of questions. This helpful review book will boost your confidence and ease your anxiety.

Topics and nursing steps

A useful supplementary study guide, this book includes 250 alternate-format questions that cover all of the topics tested on the exam — including fundamentals of nursing, medical-surgical nursing, maternal-infant nursing, pediatric nursing, and psychiatric and mental health nursing. For each type of question, you'll find the correct answer as well as clear, concise rationales for correct and incorrect answers. You'll also find the associated nursing process step, client needs category and subcategory, and cognitive level.

The convenient two-column format (with questions on the left and answers on the right) enhances your preparation process by giving you instant feedback and saves you the time of flipping to the back of the book to find the correct answer.

The review questions provided in this book will test your knowledge base and improve your test-taking skills as well as help you become familiar with the format of the new questions. All of the questions were written by nurses and approximate the real questions you'll find on the NCLEX.

NCLEX examination

Even if your examination contains only a few alternate-format questions, you can be confident that the questions in this book cover relevant information in a challenging format that can be useful even if your NCLEX examination does not include all of these new-format questions. Also, in your rush to prepare for the new-format questions, don't forget to review practice questions that follow the standard four-option, multiple-choice format. These questions will still compose the bulk of the test.

Remember that the process of testing and introducing new alternate-format questions into the NCLEX is ongoing. Because the test format is subject to change, be sure to consult the "Testing services" section of the NCSBN Web site (*www.ncsbn.org*) as your exam date nears for the most up-to-date information on the NCLEX.

You've been diligently preparing for this all-important exam for years. *NCLEX-PN: 250 New-Format Questions,* Second Edition, is the next logical extension of that sound preparation, the final resource you need to meet the challenge of passing NCLEX and moving on to the rewards of your nursing career. Good luck!

PART ONE

Fundamentals of nursing

Basic physical care

1. A nurse is caring for a client who sustained a chemical burn in his right eye. She's preparing to irrigate the eye with sterile normal saline solution. Which steps are appropriate when performing the procedure? Select all that apply.

- ☐ **1.** Tilt the client's head toward his left eye.
- ☐ **2.** Place absorbent pads in the area of the client's shoulder.
- ☐ **3.** Wash hands and put on gloves.
- ☐ **4.** Place the irrigation syringe directly on the cornea.
- ☐ **5.** Direct the solution onto the exposed conjunctival sac from the inner to outer canthus.
- ☐ **6.** Irrigate the eye for 1 minute.

Answer: 2, 3, 5

Rationale: The nurse should place absorbent pads in the area of the shoulder to prevent saturating the client's clothing and bed linens. She should also wash her hands and put on gloves to reduce the transmission of microorganisms. The solution should be directed from the inner to outer canthus of the eye to prevent contamination of the unaffected eye. The head should be tilted toward the affected (right) eye to facilitate drainage and to prevent irrigating solution from entering the left eye. The irrigation syringe should be held about 1″ (2.5 cm) above the eye to prevent injury to the cornea. In a chemical exposure, the eye should be irrigated for at least 10 minutes.

Nursing process step: Implementation

Client needs category: Physiological integrity

Client needs subcategory: Reduction of risk potential

Cognitive level: Application

---

2. A nurse is caring for a client who underwent cardiac catheterization. He starts bleeding from his left femoral access site. Identify the area where the nurse should apply pressure.

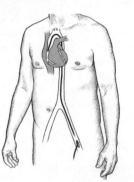

Answer:

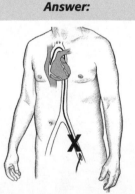

Rationale: The femoral artery is punctured approximately 2 inches above the access site.

Nursing process step: Implementation

Client needs category: Physiological integrity

Client needs subcategory: Reduction of risk potential

Cognitive level: Application

3. A nurse is preparing to leave a contact isolation room. Place the following steps in ascending chronological order as to how protective wear should be removed. Use all the options.

| 1. Remove eyewear. |
| 2. Remove gloves. |
| 3. Remove mask. |
| 4. Remove gown. |
| 5. Wash hands for a minimum of 10 seconds. |

| |
| |
| |
| |
| |

Answer:

| 2. Remove gloves. |
| 3. Remove mask. |
| 4. Remove gown. |
| 1. Remove eyewear. |
| 5. Wash hands for a minimum of 10 seconds. |

Rationale: Removal of gloves, then mask, gown, and eyewear, and then washing hands for a minimum of 10 seconds limits the possibility of contact with contaminants.

Nursing process step: Implementation

Client needs category: Safe, effective care environment

Client needs subcategory: Safety and infection control

Cognitive level: Comprehension

---

4. A client is ordered to receive a sodium phosphate enema for relief of constipation. Proper administration of the enema includes which steps? Select all that apply.

☐ **1.** Chill the solution by placing it in the refrigerator for 10 minutes.

☐ **2.** Assist the client into Sims' position.

☐ **3.** Wash hands and put on gloves.

☐ **4.** Insert the tip of the container ½" into the rectum.

☐ **5.** Allow gravity to instill the solution.

☐ **6.** Encourage the client to retain the solution for 5 to 15 minutes.

Answer: 2, 3, 6

Rationale: To administer an enema, the nurse should place the client in Sims' position or a knee-chest position. Washing hands and putting on gloves are necessary to reduce the transmission of microorganisms. To promote the effectiveness of the enema, the nurse should encourage the client to retain the solution for at least 5 minutes. The solution should be warmed rather than chilled to promote comfort. To administer the solution effectively and deliver it to the appropriate location, the nurse should insert the full length of the tip into the rectum. The nurse should compress the container to deliver the solution under positive pressure and not by gravity.

Nursing process step: Implementation

Client needs category: Physiological integrity

Client needs subcategory: Basic care and comfort

Cognitive level: Application

5. A nurse is completing the intake and output record for a client who was restarted on his regular diet after being on nothing-by-mouth status for laboratory studies. The client has had the following intake and output during the shift:

Intake: 4 oz of cranberry juice, ½ cup of oatmeal, 2 slices of toast, 8 oz of black decaffeinated coffee, tuna fish sandwich, ½ cup of fruit-flavored gelatin, 1 cup of cream of mushroom soup, 6 oz. of 1% milk, 16 oz of water

Output: 1,300 ml of urine

How many milliliters should the nurse document as the client's intake?

_____

Answer: 1380

Rationale: There are 30 ml in each ounce and 240 ml in each cup. The fluid intake for this client includes 4 oz (120 ml) of cranberry juice, 8 oz (240 ml) of coffee, ½ cup (120 ml) of fruit-flavored gelatin, 1 cup (240 ml) of cream of mushroom soup, 6 oz (180 ml) of milk, and 16 oz (480 ml) of water, for a total of 1,380.

Nursing process step: Implementation

Client needs category: Physiological integrity

Client needs subcategory: Basic care and comfort

Cognitive level: Application

6. A hospitalized client asks the nurse for "something for pain." What information is most important for the nurse to gather before administering the medication? Select all that apply.

☐ **1.** Administration time of the last dose

☐ **2.** Client's pain level on a scale of 1 to 10

☐ **3.** Type of medication the client has been taking

☐ **4.** Beeper number of the client's physician

☐ **5.** Client's most current height and weight

☐ **6.** Effectiveness of prior dose of medication

Answer: 1, 2, 3, 6

Rationale: The nurse needs to know when the last dose was administered. Some clients request pain medication earlier than is ordered by the physician. Pain, the fifth vital sign, should be assessed using a pain scale and documented in the nursing notes whenever a pain medication is given. Pain is usually reassessed about 30 minutes after the medication is given. Physicians commonly order several different types of pain medication based on the client's condition. It is important for the nurse to know which medication and which route was used to administer prior dosages. Evaluating the effectiveness of medications is also an important nursing function when managing the client's pain. Therefore, she should ask the client if the prior dose was helpful. Knowing the beeper number of the client's physician is not as important as the other choices, although most nurses know the name of their clients' physicians. Most medications aren't ordered based on the client's height, and weight. This information would have been obtained on admission.

Nursing process step: Data collection

Client needs category: Physiological integrity

Client needs subcategory: Basic care and comfort

Cognitive level: Application

7. A postoperative client has an abdominal incision. While getting out of bed, the client reports feeling a "pulling" sensation in his abdominal wound. The nurse assesses the client's wound and finds that it has separated and the abdominal organs are protruding. Which nursing interventions are most appropriate at this time? Select all that apply.

☐ **1.** Notify the client's primary physician.

☐ **2.** Cover the wound with saline-soaked sterile gauze.

☐ **3.** Give the client a dose of antibiotics.

☐ **4.** Order an abdominal binder from the supply department.

☐ **5.** Push the organs back into the abdomen.

☐ **6.** Assess the client for signs of shock.

Answer: 1, 2

Rationale: Dehiscence and evisceration are medical emergencies. The client's physician should be notified and the nurse should prepare the client for surgery. The wound and the abdominal organs should be covered with saline-soaked sterile gauze. Even though wound infection is the most common cause of dehiscence, administering antibiotics without a physician's order is not permissible. An abdominal binder may be appropriate after the client returns from the operating room. Pushing the organs back into the abdomen could cause rupture, hemorrhage, or strangulation of the bowel. Assessing for shock isn't necessary at this time.

Nursing process step: Implementation

Client needs category: Physiological integrity

Client needs subcategory: Reduction of risk potential

Cognitive level: Analysis

---

8. A nurse puts on gloves to perform a fecal occult blood test using a Hemoccult slide. Place these steps in ascending chronological order. Use all the options.

1. Allow the specimens to dry for 3 minutes.

2. Apply a drop of Hemoccult-developing solution to box A and box B on the reverse side of the slide.

3. Apply a smear of stool to box A on the slide.

4. Apply a smear of stool from another part of the specimen to box B on the slide.

5. Apply a drop of Hemoccult-developing solution to each control dot on the reverse side of the slide.

6. Evaluate the results; remove gloves; wash hands.

Answer:

3. Apply a smear of stool to box A on the slide.

4. Apply a smear of stool from another part of the specimen to box B on the slide.

1. Allow the specimens to dry for 3 minutes.

5. Apply a drop of Hemoccult-developing solution to each control dot on the reverse side of the slide.

2. Apply a drop of Hemoccult-developing solution to box A and box B on the reverse side of the slide.

6. Evaluate the results; remove gloves; and wash hands.

Rationale: Upon receiving the specimen, using a wooden applicator, smear a small amount of stool in box A and a small amount of stool from a different part of the specimen in box B. The expiration date on the developer bottle should be checked and the bottle discarded if expired. A blue reaction after 30 to 60 seconds indicates a positive result.

Nursing process step: Implementation

Client needs category: Health promotion and maintenance

Client needs subcategory: None

Cognitive level: Application

9. A client suffers a broken leg as a result of a car accident and is taken to the emergency department. A plaster cast is applied. Before discharge, the nurse provides the client with instructions regarding cast care. Which instructions are most appropriate? Select all that apply.

☐ **1.** Support the wet cast with pillows until it dries.

☐ **2.** Use a hair dryer to speed the drying process.

☐ **3.** Use the fingertips when moving the wet cast.

☐ **4.** Apply powder to the inside of the cast after it dries.

☐ **5.** Notify the physician if itching occurs under the cast.

☐ **6.** Avoid putting straws or hangers inside the cast.

Answer: 1, 6

Rationale: Supporting the wet cast with pillows prevents the cast from changing shape and interfering with the alignment of the fractured bone. The nurse should instruct the client not to place sharp objects, such as straws or hangers, down the inside of the cast to avoid the risk of impairing the skin and causing infection. Using a hair dryer is not advised because it dries the cast unevenly, can cause burns to the tissue, and can crack the cast, causing poor alignment to the injured bone. The palms, not the fingertips, should be used when handling the wet cast because fingertips can dent the cast, thus causing pressure points that can affect the skin's integrity. Powder should not be used because it can cake under the cast. Itching is a common occurrence with casts because the skin cells are unable to slough as they normally would and the dry skin causes itching. Normally, the physician is not called for this problem.

Nursing process step: Implementation

Client needs category: Physiological integrity

Client needs subcategory: Basic care and comfort

Cognitive level: Comprehension

---

10. A nurse is caring for a client with a hiatal hernia. The client complains of abdominal and sternal pain after eating. The pain makes it difficult for the client to sleep. Which instructions should the nurse stress when teaching this client? Select all that apply.

☐ **1.** Avoid constrictive clothing.

☐ **2.** Lie down for 30 minutes after eating.

☐ **3.** Decrease intake of caffeine and spicy foods.

☐ **4.** Eat three meals per day.

☐ **5.** Sleep in semi-Fowler position.

☐ **6.** Maintain a normal body weight.

Answer: 1, 3, 5, 6

Rationale: To reduce gastric reflux, the nurse should instruct the client to avoid constrictive clothing, caffeine, and spicy foods; remain upright for 2 hours after eating; eat small, frequent meals; sleep with his upper body elevated; and lose weight, if obese.

Nursing process step: Implementation

Client needs category: Physiological integrity

Client needs subcategory: Basic care and comfort

Cognitive level: Application

11. A client is admitted to the hospital from an extended care facility with a stage 3 pressure ulcer. Identify the deepest layer of tissue involved in this diagnosis.

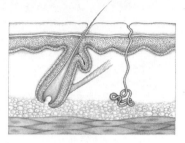

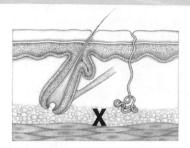

Rationale: A stage 3 pressure ulcer is full-thickness skin loss. Therefore, the deepest layer involved is the subcutaneous tissue level. The epidermis and dermis are involved in stage 1 ulceration.

Nursing process step: Data collection

Client needs category: Physiological integrity

Client needs subcategory: Physiological adaptation

Cognitive level: Application

---

12. A nurse investigates the smell of smoke in the hallway of a long-term care unit. She enters a client's room and finds the wastebasket is on fire. The nurse takes immediate action. Place the nurse's actions in proper ascending chronological order. Use all the options.

1. Trigger the alarm.
2. Extinguish the fire.
3. Rescue the client.
4. Confine the fire.

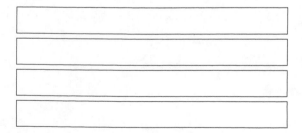

Answer:

3. Rescue the client.
1. Trigger the alarm.
4. Confine the fire.
2. Extinguish the fire.

Rationale: Based on the RACE (Rescue, Alarm, Confine, Extinguish) mnemonic, the nurse's first priority is the client's safety. The second need is to summon help in the emergency. Next, the nurse can attempt to confine then extinguish the fire.

Nursing process step: Implementation

Client needs category: Safe, effective care environment

Client needs subcategory: Safety and infection control

Cognitive level: Comprehension

Basic psychosocial needs

1. A nurse is caring for a client who's disoriented to time, place, and person and is attempting to get out of bed and pull out an I.V. line that's supplying hydration and antibiotics. The client has a vest restraint and bilateral soft wrist restraints. Which actions by the nurse would be appropriate? Select all that apply.

☐ **1.** Recheck and document the behavior that requires continued use of restraints.

☐ **2.** Tie the restraints in quick-release knots.

☐ **3.** Tie the restraints to the side rails of the bed.

☐ **4.** Ask the client if he needs to go to the bathroom, and provide range-of-motion (ROM) exercises every 2 hours.

☐ **5.** Position the vest restraints so that the straps are crossed in the back.

Answer: 1, 2, 4

Rationale: The client must be checked frequently to determine whether he's ready to have the restraints removed. The information should also be documented. Restraints should be tied in knots that can be released quickly and easily. Toileting and ROM exercises should be performed every 2 hours while a client is in restraints. Restraints should never be secured to side rails because doing so can cause injury if the side rail is lowered without untying the restraint. A vest restraint should be positioned so the straps cross in front of the client, not in the back.

Nursing process step: Implementation

Client needs category: Safe, effective care environment

Client needs subcategory: Safety and infection control

Cognitive level: Application

---

2. A client has just been diagnosed with terminal cancer and is being transferred to home hospice care. The client's daughter tells the nurse, "I don't know what to say to my mother if she asks me if she's going to die." Which responses by the nurse would be appropriate? Select all that apply.

☐ **1.** "Tell your mother not to worry; she still has some time left."

☐ **2.** "Let's talk about your mother's illness and how it will progress."

☐ **3.** "You sound like you have some questions about your mother dying. Let's talk about that."

☐ **4.** "Don't worry. Hospice will take care of your mother."

☐ **5.** "Tell me how you're feeling about your mother dying."

Answer: 2, 3, 5

Rationale: Conveying information and providing clear communication can alleviate fears and strengthen the individual's sense of control. Encouraging verbalization of feelings helps build a therapeutic relationship based on trust and reduces anxiety. Telling the daughter not to worry ignores her feelings and discourages further communication. Having her tell her mother not to worry has the same effect on their communication.

Nursing process step: Implementation

Client needs category: Psychosocial integrity

Client needs subcategory: None

Cognitive level: Analysis

3. While providing care to a 26-year-old married female, a nurse notes multiple ecchymotic areas on her arms and trunk. The color of the ecchymotic areas ranges from blue to purple to yellow. When asked by the nurse how she got these bruises, the client responds, "Oh, I tripped." How should the nurse respond? Select all that apply.

- ☐ **1.** Document the client's statement and complete a body map indicating the size, color, shape, location, and type of injuries.
- ☐ **2.** Contact the local authorities to report suspicions of abuse.
- ☐ **3.** Assist the client in developing a safety plan for times of increased violence.
- ☐ **4.** Call the client's husband to arrange a meeting to discuss the situation.
- ☐ **5.** Tell the client that she needs to leave the abusive situation as soon as possible.
- ☐ **6.** Provide the client with telephone numbers of local shelters and safe houses.

Answer: 1, 3, 6

Rationale: The nurse should objectively document her assessment findings. A detailed description of physical findings of abuse in the medical record is essential if legal action is pursued. All women suspected to be victims of abuse should be counseled on a safety plan, which consists of recognizing escalating violence within the family and formulating a plan to exit quickly. The nurse should not report this suspicion of abuse because the client is a competent adult who has the right to self-determination. Nurses do, however, have a duty to report cases of actual or suspected abuse in children or elderly clients. Contacting the client's husband without her consent violates confidentiality. The nurse should respond to the client in a nonthreatening manner that promotes trust, rather than ordering her to break off her relationship.

Nursing process step: Implementation

Client needs category: Psychosocial integrity

Client needs subcategory: None

Cognitive level: Analysis

---

4. A nurse is caring for a client who's terminally ill. Place the symptoms of the five stages of death and dying described by Elisabeth Kübler-Ross in ascending chronological order. Use all the options.

| **1.** Negotiating, new interest in healthful behaviors |
| **2.** Withdrawal, refusal to discuss health issues |
| **3.** Calmness, honesty, involved in care management decisions |
| **4.** Irritability, complaining, adversarial |
| **5.** Loss, grief, intense sadness |

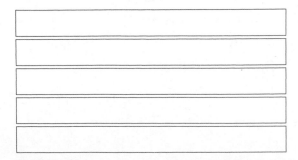

Answer:

| **2.** Withdrawal, refusal to discuss health issues |
| **4.** Irritability, complaining, adversarial |
| **1.** Negotiating, new interest in healthful behaviors |
| **5.** Loss, grief, intense sadness |
| **3.** Calmness, honesty, involved in care management decisions |

Rationale: According to Kübler-Ross, the five stages of death and dying are denial and isolation, anger, bargaining, depression, and acceptance.

Nursing process step: Data collection

Client needs category: Psychosocial integrity

Client needs category: None

Cognitive level: Analysis

5. A 26-year-old client with chronic renal failure was recently told by his physician that he's a poor candidate for a transplant because of chronic uncontrolled hypertension and diabetes mellitus. Now, the client tells the nurse, "I want to go off dialysis. I'd rather not live than be on this treatment for the rest of my life." Which responses by the nurse are appropriate? Select all that apply.

☐ **1.** Take a seat next to the client and sit quietly to reflect on what was said.

☐ **2.** Say to the client, "We all have days when we don't feel like going on."

☐ **3.** Leave the room to allow the client privacy to collect his thoughts.

☐ **4.** Say to the client, "You're feeling upset about the news you got about a transplant."

☐ **5.** Say to the client, "The treatments are only 3 days a week. You can live with that."

Answer: 1, 4

Rationale: Silence is a therapeutic communication technique that allows the nurse and client to reflect on what has taken place or been said. By waiting quietly and attentively, the nurse encourages the client to initiate and maintain conversation. By reflecting the client's implied feelings, the nurse promotes communication. Using such platitudes as "We all have days when we don't feel like going on" fails to address the client's needs. The nurse should not leave the client alone because he may harm himself. Reminding the client of the treatment frequency doesn't address his feelings.

Nursing process step: Implementation

Client needs category: Psychosocial integrity

Client needs subcategory: None

Cognitive level: Analysis

---

6. A nurse is collecting data on a newly admitted client. When filling out the family assessment, who should the nurse consider to be a part of the client's family? Select all that apply.

☐ **1.** People related by blood or marriage

☐ **2.** People whom the client views as family

☐ **3.** People who live in the same house

☐ **4.** People who the nurse thinks are important to the client

☐ **5.** People who live in the same house with the same racial background as the client

☐ **6.** People who provide for the physical and emotional needs of the client

Answer: 2, 6

Rationale: When providing care to a client, the nurse should consider family members to be all the people whom the client views as family. Family members may also include those people who provide for the physical and emotional needs of the client. The traditional definition of a family has changed and may include people not related by blood or marriage, those of a different racial background, and those who may not live in the same house as the client. Family members are defined by the client, not by the nurse.

Nursing process step: Data collection

Client needs category: Health promotion and maintenance

Client needs subcategory: None

Cognitive level: Analysis

7. A nurse is caring for a client whose cultural background is different from her own. Which actions are appropriate for the nurse? Select all that apply.

☐ **1.** Consider that nonverbal cues such as eye contact may have a different meaning in different cultures.

☐ **2.** Respect the client's cultural beliefs.

☐ **3.** Ask the client if he has cultural or religious requirements that should be considered in his care.

☐ **4.** Explain the nurse's beliefs so that the client will understand the differences.

☐ **5.** Understand that all cultures experience pain in the same way.

Answer: 1, 2, 3

Rationale: Nonverbal cues may have different meanings in different cultures. In one culture, eye contact is a sign of disrespect; in another, eye contact shows respect and attentiveness. The nurse should always respect the client's cultural beliefs and ask if he has cultural requirements. This may include food choices or restrictions, body coverings, or time for prayer. The nurse should attempt to understand the client's culture; it is not the client's responsibility to understand the nurse's culture. The nurse should never impose her own beliefs on her clients. Culture influences a client's experience with pain. For example, in one culture pain may be openly expressed whereas in another culture it may be quietly endured.

Nursing process step: Planning

Client needs category: Psychosocial integrity

Client needs subcategory: None

Cognitive level: Analysis

---

8. A nurse is caring for a 45-year-old married woman who has undergone hemicolectomy for colon cancer. The woman has two children. Which concepts about families should the nurse keep in mind when providing care for this client? Select all that apply.

☐ **1.** Illness in one family member can affect all members.

☐ **2.** Family roles don't change because of illness.

☐ **3.** A family member may have more than one role at a time in a family.

☐ **4.** Children typically aren't affected by adult illness.

☐ **5.** The effects of an illness on a family depend on the stage of the family's life cycle.

☐ **6.** Changes in sleeping and eating patterns may be signs of stress in a family.

Answer: 1, 3, 5, 6

Rationale: Illness in one family member can affect all family members, even children. Each member of a family may have several roles to perform. A middle-aged woman, for example, may have the roles of mother, wage-earner, wife, and housekeeper. Families move through certain predictable life cycles (such as birth of a baby, a growing family, adult children leaving home, and grandparenting). The impact of illness on the family depends on the stage of the life cycle, as family members take on different roles and the family structure changes. Illness produces stress in families; changes in eating and sleeping patterns are signs of stress. When one family member can't fulfill a role because of illness, the roles of the other family members are affected.

Nursing process step: Implementation

Client needs category: Health promotion and maintenance

Client needs subcategory: None

Cognitive level: Analysis

9. Every client admitted to the hospital must receive information about advance directives. Which statements are true about advance directives? Select all that apply.

☐ **1.** Every person must complete an advance directive upon admission.

☐ **2.** An advance directive includes a living will or a power of health care attorney.

☐ **3.** An advance directive is a legal document.

☐ **4.** An advance directive must be notarized.

☐ **5.** An advance directive should be included with the client's chart.

☐ **6.** An advance directive conveys the client's directions about his health care upon loss of capacity.

Rationale: An advance directive is a legal document used as a guideline for life-sustaining medical care of a client with an advanced disease or disability who can no longer indicate his own wishes. An advance directive includes a living will, which instructs the physician to administer no life-sustaining treatment, and a durable power of attorney for health care, which names another person to act on the client's behalf for medical decisions. The client isn't required to complete an advance directive; however, by law, the explanation of the document and the opportunity to complete it are given to every client. An advance directive is best when notarized, but is considered valid upon the signature of two disinterested witnesses. It should be included with the patient's chart.

Nursing process step: Data collection

Client needs category: Safe, effective care environment

Client needs subcategory: Coordinated care

Cognitive level: Comprehension

---

10. A nurse is working with the family of a client who has Alzheimer's disease. The nurse notes that the client's spouse is too exhausted to continue providing care all alone. The adult children live too far away to provide relief on a weekly basis. Which nursing interventions would be helpful? Select all that apply.

☐ **1.** Calling a family meeting to tell the absent children that they must participate in caregiving

☐ **2.** Suggesting the spouse seek psychological counseling to help cope with exhaustion

☐ **3.** Recommending community resources for adult day care and respite care

☐ **4.** Encouraging the spouse to talk about the difficulties involved in caring for a loved one

☐ **5.** Asking whether friends or church members can help with errands or provide short periods of relief

☐ **6.** Recommending that the client be placed in a long-term care facility

Rationale: Many community services exist for Alzheimer's clients and their families. Encouraging use of these resources may make it possible for the client to stay at home and to alleviate the spouse's exhaustion. The nurse can also support the caregiver by urging her to talk about the difficulties she's facing in caring for a spouse. Friends and church members may be able to help provide care to the client, allowing the caregiver time for rest, exercise, or an enjoyable activity. A family meeting to tell the children to participate more would probably be ineffective and may evoke anger or guilt. Counseling may be helpful, but it wouldn't alleviate the caregiver's physical exhaustion and wouldn't address the client's immediate needs. A long-term care facility is not an option until the family is ready to make that decision.

Nursing process step: Implementation

Client needs category: Psychosocial integrity

Client needs subcategory: None

Cognitive level: Analysis

Medication and I.V. administration

1. A client has just had total hip replacement surgery. The physician orders heparin 8,000 units to be administered subcutaneously. The label on the heparin vial reads: heparin 10,000 units/ml. How many milliliters of heparin should the nurse draw up in the syringe to administer the correct dose?

_____

Rationale: The following formula is used to calculate drug dosages:

Dose on hand/Quantity on hand = Dose desired/X

In this example, the equation is as follows:

$$10{,}000 \text{ units/ml} = 8{,}000 \text{ units}/X$$

$$X = 0.8 \text{ ml.}$$

Nursing process step: Implementation

Client needs category: Physiological integrity

Client needs subcategory: Pharmacological therapies

Cognitive level: Application

2. After laparoscopic cholecystectomy, a client complains of pain and nausea. The nurse is preparing meperidine hydrochloride (Demerol) 75 mg and promethazine hydrochloride (Phenergan) 12.5 mg to be administered I.M. in the same syringe. If the label on the Demerol reads 50 mg/ml and the label on the Phenergan reads 25 mg/ml, how many milliliters should the nurse have in the syringe after the correct doses are drawn up?

_____

Rationale: Use the following formula:

Dose on hand/Quantity on hand = Dose desired/X

In this example, the formula is as follows:

$$50 \text{ mg/ml} = 75 \text{ mg}/X$$

$$X = 1.5 \text{ ml.}$$

The formula for calculating the amount of Phenergan is as follows:

$$25 \text{ mg/ml} = 12.5 \text{ mg}/X$$

$$X = 0.5 \text{ ml.}$$

To calculate the total milliliters that should be drawn up in the syringe, the nurse adds the quantity of Demerol and the quantity of Phenergan, as follows:

1.5 ml + 0.5 ml = 2 ml total drawn up in the syringe.

Nursing process step: Implementation

Client needs category: Physiological integrity

Client needs subcategory: Pharmacological therapies

Cognitive level: Application

3. A nurse is reinforcing a teaching plan with a client who's prescribed enalapril maleate (Vasotec) for treatment of hypertension. Which instructions would the nurse expect to see included in the teaching plan? Select all that apply.

☐ **1.** Instruct the client to avoid salt substitutes.

☐ **2.** Tell the client that light-headedness is a common adverse effect that need not be reported.

☐ **3.** Inform the client that he may have a sore throat for the first few days of therapy.

☐ **4.** Tell the client that blood tests will be necessary every 3 weeks for 2 months and periodically thereafter.

☐ **5.** Advise the client to report facial swelling or difficulty breathing immediately.

☐ **6.** Inform the client not to change position suddenly to minimize orthostatic hypotension.

Answer: 1, 5, 6

Rationale: When teaching a client about enalapril, the nurse should tell him to avoid salt substitutes because these products may contain potassium, which can cause light-headedness and syncope. Facial swelling or difficulty breathing should be reported immediately. The drug may cause angioedema, which would require discontinuation of the drug. The client should also be advised to change position slowly to minimize orthostatic hypotension. The nurse should tell the client to report light-headedness, especially in the first few days of therapy, so dosage adjustments can be made. The client should report signs of infection, such as sore throat and fever, because the drug may decrease the client's white blood cell (WBC) count. This effect is generally seen within 3 months, so WBC and differential counts should be performed periodically.

Nursing process step: Planning

Client needs category: Physiological integrity

Client needs subcategory: Pharmacological therapies

Cognitive level: Application

---

4. A nurse is administering ampicillin (Polycillin) 125 mg I.M. every 6 hours to a 10-kg child with a respiratory tract infection. The drug label reads, "The recommended dosage for a client weighing less than 40 kg is 25 to 50 mg/kg/day I.M. or I.V. in equally divided doses at 6- to 8-hour intervals." The drug concentration is 125 mg/5 ml. Which nursing interventions are appropriate at this time? Select all that apply.

☐ **1.** Draw up 10 ml of ampicillin to administer.

☐ **2.** Administer the medication at 1000, 1400, 1800, and 2200.

☐ **3.** Assess the client for allergies to penicillin.

☐ **4.** Administer the medication because it's within the dosing recommendations.

☐ **5.** Question the physician about the order because it's more than the recommended dosage.

☐ **6.** Obtain a sputum culture before administering the medication.

Answer: 3, 4, 6

Rationale: Because ampicillin is a penicillin antibiotic, the client should be assessed for allergy to penicillin before the medication is administered. The dose of ampicillin is within the recommended dosage range for a 10-kg client: 50 mg/kg × 10 kg = 500 mg. A dose of 500 mg divided by 4 (given every 6 hours) = 125 mg, which is within the recommended range. Cultures, if ordered, should be obtained before antibiotics are given. The nurse should draw up 5 ml to administer the correct dose, according to the concentration on the label. The 1000, 1400, 1800, and 2200 dosing schedule is in 4-hour intervals and shouldn't be used because the recommended dosing is in 6- to 8-hour intervals.

Nursing process step: Implementation

Client needs category: Physiological integrity

Client needs subcategory: Pharmacological therapies

Cognitive level: Analysis

5. A nurse is using the Z-track method of I.M. injection to administer iron dextran to a client with iron deficiency anemia. Which techniques should the nurse use to give this injection? Select all that apply.

- ☐ **1.** Confirm the client's identity before administering the iron dextran.
- ☐ **2.** Inject the iron dextran into the deltoid muscle.
- ☐ **3.** Change the needle after drawing up the iron dextran.
- ☐ **4.** Before inserting the needle, displace the skin laterally by pulling it away from the injection site.
- ☐ **5.** Inject the iron dextran after aspirating for a blood return.
- ☐ **6.** After removing the needle, massage the injection site.

Answer: 1, 3, 4, 5

Rationale: Before administering any medication, the nurse confirms the client's identity. After drawing up iron dextran, she removes the first needle and attaches a second needle to prevent tracking the medication through the subcutaneous tissue when the needle is inserted. To administer the injection by Z-track method, the nurse first displaces the skin laterally by pulling it away from the injection site. The nurse should aspirate for a blood return before administering iron dextran; if no blood appears, the medication may be injected. Iron dextran should be administered into the large dorsogluteal muscle only. After injecting iron dextran, the nurse shouldn't massage the site because this could force the medication into the subcutaneous tissue.

Nursing process step: Implementation

Client needs category: Physiological integrity

Client needs subcategory: Pharmacological therapies

Cognitive level: Application

---

6. The nurse is preparing to administer regular insulin 4 units to a client with type 1 diabetes mellitus. Which equipment does the nurse need to perform the injection? Select all that apply.

- ☐ **1.** Medication administration record
- ☐ **2.** Nursing assessment sheet
- ☐ **3.** 27-gauge, ½" needle
- ☐ **4.** 22-gauge, ½" needle
- ☐ **5.** 27-gauge, 1" needle
- ☐ **6.** 22-gauge 1" needle

Answer: 1, 3

Rationale: To administer medication, the nurse needs the medication administration record to verify the correct client, medication, dose, time, and route. A subcutaneous injection, such as insulin, is administered with a 25-gauge to 27-gauge, ⅝" to ½" needle. The nursing assessment sheet isn't necessary for administering insulin. A 22-gauge needle is too large for a subcutaneous injection. A 1" needle may deliver the medication into muscle rather than subcutaneous tissue.

Nursing process step: Implementation

Client needs category: Physiological integrity

Client needs subcategory: Pharmacological therapies

Cognitive level: Application

7. A nurse is administering insulin to a client with type 1 diabetes mellitus. Identify the tissue layer where the tip of the needle should be placed to deliver this medication to the proper tissue.

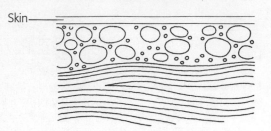

Answer:

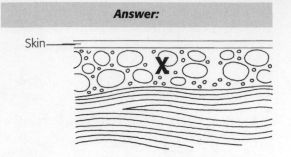

Rationale: Insulin is administered by subcutaneous injection. The tip of the needle should be in the subcutaneous tissue.

Nursing process step: Implementation

Client needs category: Physiological integrity

Client needs subcategory: Pharmacological therapies

Cognitive level: Comprehension

---

8. A client with heart failure is ordered 60 mg of furosemide (Lasix) P.O. daily. Because the client has difficulty swallowing, an oral solution is ordered. The solution dispensed from the pharmacy has a concentration of 40 mg/5 ml. How many milliliters should the nurse administer?

Answer: 7.5

Rationale: Use the following formula:

Dose on hand/Quantity on hand = Dose desired/X

40 mg/5 ml = 60 mg/X

$X = 7.5$ ml.

Nursing process step: Implementation

Client needs category: Physiological integrity

Client needs subcategory: Pharmacological therapies

Cognitive level: Application

9. A client with an I.V. line in place complains of pain at the insertion site. Assessment of the site reveals a vein that is red, warm, and hard. Which actions should the nurse take? Select all that apply.

- ☐ **1.** Slow the infusion rate while notifying the prescriber.
- ☐ **2.** Discontinue the infusion at the affected site.
- ☐ **3.** Request restart of the infusion in an I.V. site distal to the discontinued I.V. site.
- ☐ **4.** Check the client for skin sloughing.
- ☐ **5.** Apply warm soaks to the I.V. site.
- ☐ **6.** Document the examination, the nurse's actions, and the client's responses.

Rationale: Redness, warmth, pain, and a hard, cordlike vein at the I.V. insertion site suggest that the client has phlebitis. The nurse should discontinue the I.V. line and insert a new I.V. catheter proximal to or above the discontinued I.V. site or in the other arm. Skin sloughing is associated with extravasation of certain toxic medications and should be included in the assessment and actions. Applying warm soaks to the site reduces inflammation. The nurse should document her assessment, actions taken, and the client's response. When phlebitis is present, slowing the infusion rate won't reduce the phlebitis. Restarting the infusion at a site distal to the phlebitis may contribute to the inflammation.

Nursing process step: Implementation

Client needs category: Physiological integrity

Client needs subcategory: Pharmacological therapies

Cognitive level: Application

---

10. A nurse is administering an I.M. injection into the vastus lateralis muscle. Identify the area where the nurse will inject the medication.

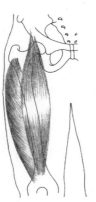

Answer:

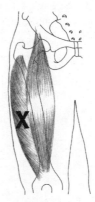

Rationale: The vastus lateralis is an I.M. injection site located in the middle third of the outer aspect of the thigh, from a handbreadth below the greater trochanter to a handbreadth above the knee.

Nursing process step: Implementation

Client needs category: Physiological integrity

Client needs subcategory: Pharmacological therapies

Cognitive level: Application

11. A physician orders amoxicillin (Amoxil) 250 mg P.O. (by mouth) t.i.d. for a client. Amoxicillin 125 mg/tsp is available. How many tsp must the nurse administer?

Answer: 2

Rationale: Use the following equation:

$$1 \text{ tsp}/125 \text{ mg} \times 250 \text{ mg}/1 \text{ dose}$$

$$250 \text{ tsp}/125 \text{ dose} = 2 \text{ tsp/dose}.$$

Nursing process step: Intervention

Client needs category: Physiological integrity

Client needs subcategory: Pharmacological therapies

Cognitive level: Application

---

12. A client on hemodialysis is prescribed cephalexin (Keflex) 500 mg P.O. (by mouth) every 6 hours for a group A beta-hemolytic streptococcal infection. The client states that he can't swallow the large pills and requests a liquid dose. The suspension is available in 250 mg/5 ml. The nurse knows that which statements about this order are true? Select all that apply.

- ☐ **1.** The maximum oral dosage of cephalexin for an adult is 4 g daily.

- ☐ **2.** Hypersensitivity to penicillin and cephalosporin is a contraindication to use of this drug.

- ☐ **3.** The dosage prescribed for the client is within an acceptable range for a client on hemodialysis.

- ☐ **4.** Adverse effects of nausea and anorexia may be relieved by taking the drug with food or milk.

- ☐ **5.** Stevens-Johnson syndrome is an adverse effect of this drug.

- ☐ **6.** Diarrhea is a common but not serious adverse reaction to this drug.

Answer: 1, 4

Rationale: The maximum oral dosage of cephalexin is 4 g daily; higher dosages must be administered I.V. Although food delays the absorption of cephalexin, it doesn't decrease it, so nausea and anorexia may be relieved by taking the drug with food or milk. A hypersensitivity to penicillin isn't a contraindication for use of cephalexin; however, use caution when administering this drug because of the cross-reactivity of cephalosporins such as cephalexin with penicillin. All cephalosporins would be contraindicated if the client had an allergy to any one of them. A client with impaired renal function and reduced creatinine clearance would not be prescribed a usual adult dosage of cephalexin as listed above. The dosage amount or frequency of administration would be lowered to adjust for delayed clearance. A red or maculopapular rash might occur with this drug, but Stevens-Johnson syndrome isn't a known reaction. Diarrhea can be a serious adverse effect, especially if found to be symptomatic of pseudomembranous colitis, which can be life-threatening.

Nursing process step: Planning

Client needs category: Physiological integrity

Client needs subcategory: Pharmacological therapies

Cognitive level: Analysis

13. A nurse transcribes the following physician's order onto the client's medication record:

March 15, 2006   1630
Administer 10 gtt of timolol maleate (Timoptic)
   ophthalmic solution AU daily.
John Bloom, MD

Which components of the medication order should the nurse question? Select all that apply.

☐ **1.** Number of drops

☐ **2.** Route

☐ **3.** Type of medication

☐ **4.** Signature

☐ **5.** Frequency of administration

☐ **6.** Date

Answer: 1, 2

Rationale: To ensure that medication errors don't occur, it's important for the nurse to follow the six rights to safe medication administration: right drug, right dose, right route, right time, right client, and right documentation. The number of drops is too great to be instilled into the eye. The medication wouldn't be effective because the dose is too large and would run out. Normally, the physician orders 1 or 2 drops to be instilled into the eye. The correct abbreviation for both eyes is OU. As the order is written, the eye medication would be administered in both ears (AU).

Nursing process step: Evaluation

Client needs category: Safe, effective care environment

Client needs subcategory: Safety and infection control

Cognitive level: Analysis

Basic physical assessment

1. An adolescent client seeks medical attention because of a sore throat and probable mononucleosis. The nurse palpates the client's submandibular lymph nodes for enlargement. Identify the area where the nurse should palpate to best feel these nodes.

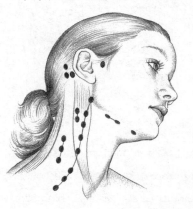

Answer:

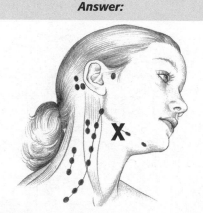

Rationale: The submandibular lymph nodes are located beneath the mandible, or lower jaw, halfway to the chin. These nodes may be enlarged in a client with a throat infection or mononucleosis.

Nursing process step: Data collection

Client needs category: Physiological integrity

Client needs subcategory: Physiological adaptation

Cognitive level: Knowledge

2. A client is hospitalized with pneumonia for 2 days. After reading the documentation below, what's the nurse's assessment of the arterial blood gas results?

4/16/2006 1530	
Arterial blood gases	
pH	7.48
Pco_2	32 mm Hg
Po_2	88 mm Hg
Sao_2	90%
HCO_3^-	24 mEq/L

☐ **1.** Respiratory acidosis

☐ **2.** Respiratory alkalosis

☐ **3.** Metabolic acidosis

☐ **4.** Metabolic alkalosis

Answer: 2

Rationale: The client is in respiratory alkalosis. The pH is increased, meaning alkalosis, not acidosis. The Pco_2 is abnormal (decreased), showing respiratory involvement, not metabolic. The HCO_3^- is normal and the Po_2 is decreased, demonstrating hypoxemia. This interpretation correlates with the initial stages of respiratory distress with an increased respiratory rate.

Nursing process step: Data collection

Client needs category: Physiological integrity

Client needs subcategory: Physiological adaptation

Cognitive level: Application

---

3. A client is admitted to the hospital for a fractured hip. He has a history of aortic stenosis. Identify the area where the nurse should place the stethoscope to best hear the murmur.

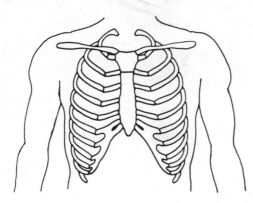

Answer:

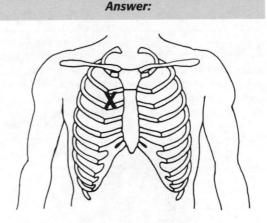

Rationale: The murmur of aortic stenosis is low-pitched, rough, and rasping. It's loudest in the second intercostal space, to the right of the sternum.

Nursing process step: Data collection

Client needs category: Health promotion and maintenance

Client needs subcategory: None

Cognitive level: Application

4. A nurse is collecting data on a client who has a rash on his chest and upper arms. Which questions should the nurse ask in order to obtain more information about the client's rash? Select all that apply.

☐ **1.** "When did the rash start?"

☐ **2.** "Are you allergic to any medications, foods, or pollen?"

☐ **3.** "How old are you?"

☐ **4.** "What have you been using to treat the rash?"

☐ **5.** "Have you traveled outside of the country?"

☐ **6.** "Do you smoke cigarettes or drink alcohol?"

Rationale: Finding out when the rash first appeared helps the physician make a diagnosis and determine the rash's stage in the disease process. Obtaining an allergy history is necessary because rashes related to allergies can occur when a client changes medications, eats new foods, or has contact with allergens in the air (such as pollen). How the client has been treating the rash is important because topical ointments and oral medications may make the rash worse. Travel outside of the country exposes the client to foreign foods and environments that can contribute to the onset of a rash. The client's age and smoking or drinking habits have no real value in determining the cause of the rash.

Nursing process step: Data collection

Client needs category: Physiological integrity

Client needs subcategory: Physiological adaptation

Cognitive level: Application

---

5. A client comes to the clinic complaining of hearing loss. The nurse performs Weber's test to assess the client's ability to hear. Identify the location where the nurse should place the tuning fork to perform this test.

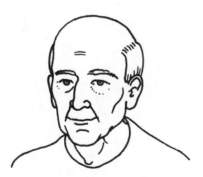

Answer:

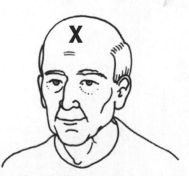

Rationale: To perform Weber's test, the tuning fork should be struck and then placed on the midline of the head. Weber's test determines if sound is heard equally in both ears. If the client hears the sound louder in one ear, he probably has unequal hearing loss that requires further intervention.

Nursing process step: Data collection

Client needs category: Health promotion and maintenance

Client needs subcategory: None

Cognitive level: Knowledge

6. A nurse realizes that as a client experiences neurologic deterioration, symptoms of "disorientation" usually occur sequentially. Place the following symptoms in ascending chronological order. Use all the options.

1.	Disoriented to familiar people
2.	Disoriented to time
3.	Disoriented to self
4.	Disoriented to place

Answer:

2.	Disoriented to time
4.	Disoriented to place
1.	Disoriented to familiar people
3.	Disoriented to self

Rationale: As a client's neurologic condition begins to deteriorate, a particular progression appears. Generally, the initial stage of disorientation is to time followed by disorientation to place. As the neurologic impairment worsens, disorientation to familiar people and then disorientation to self will occur.

Nursing process step: Data collection

Client needs category: Physiological integrity

Client needs subcategory: Physiologic adaptation

Cognitive level: Application

---

7. A client is admitted with a diagnosis of new-onset atrial fibrillation. To obtain an accurate pulse count, the nurse counts the apical heart rate. Identify the area where the nurse should place the stethoscope to best hear the apical rate.

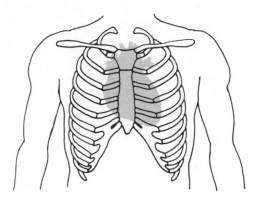

Answer:

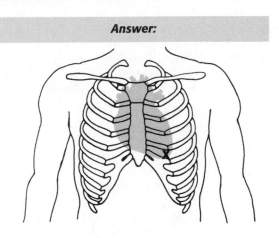

Rationale: The apical heart rate is best heard at the point of maximal impulse, which is generally in the fifth intercostal space at the midclavicular line.

Nursing process step: Data collection

Client needs category: Health promotion and maintenance

Client needs subcategory: None

Cognitive level: Application

8. An elderly client who is 5'4" and weighs 145 lb is admitted to the long-term care facility. The admitting nurse takes this report: The client sits for long periods in his wheelchair and has bowel and bladder incontinence. He is able to feed himself and has a fair appetite, eating best at breakfast and poorly thereafter. He doesn't have family members living nearby and is often noted to be crying to sleep. He also frequently requires large doses of sedatives. Which factors place the client at risk for developing a pressure ulcer? Select all that apply.

☐ **1.** Weight

☐ **2.** Incontinence

☐ **3.** Sitting for long periods of time

☐ **4.** Sedation

☐ **5.** Crying

☐ **6.** Eating poorly at lunch and dinner

Answer: 2, 3, 4

Rationale: Incontinence, inactivity, immobility, and sedation are all risk factors for developing pressure ulcers. The client's weight and poor eating habits at lunch and dinner aren't directly related to the risk of developing pressure ulcers, but a calorie count should be taken to see if the client is getting adequate calories and fluids because poor nutrition can contribute to pressure ulcers. The fact that the client cries and may be depressed has no direct bearing on this client's risk of developing a pressure ulcer. However, clients with depression are commonly not as active, so his activity levels should be monitored closely.

Nursing process step: Data collection

Client needs category: Physiological integrity

Client needs subcategory: Reduction of risk potential

Cognitive level: Analysis

---

9. A nurse finds a client lying on the floor of the hospital corridor. After determining unconsciousness, breathlessness, and providing two ventilations, the nurse checks the client's carotid artery for a pulse. Identify the area where the nurse can best palpate the carotid pulse.

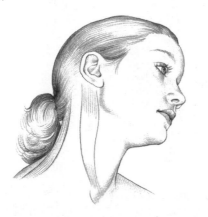

Answer:

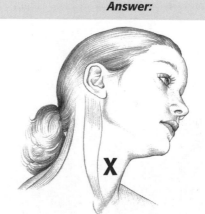

Rationale: The carotid artery is located in the neck in the groove between the trachea and the sternocleidomastoid muscle. It's the artery of choice for determining a pulse in this situation because it's usually the most accessible.

Nursing process step: Data collection

Client needs category: Physiological integrity

Client needs subcategory: Physiological adaptation

Cognitive level: Knowledge

10. A client with diabetes comes to the clinic for medical attention because of numbness and tingling in his lower extremities. The nurse obtains the client's vital signs and palpates the dorsalis pedis pulse. Identify the area where the nurse places her fingers to palpate the pedal pulse.

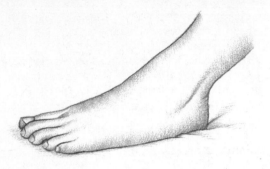

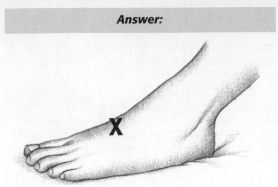

Rationale: The pedal pulse is located on the top portion of the foot. Because clients with diabetes have complications related to circulation in the lower extremities, health care providers should palpate pedal pulses and check capillary refill.

Nursing process step: Data collection

Client needs category: Health promotion and maintenance

Client needs subcategory: None

Cognitive level: Knowledge

---

11. A client comes to the emergency department seeking medical attention for severe pain in the area of the appendix. Identify the area where the nurse would expect the pain to localize.

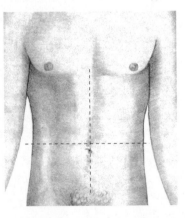

Answer:

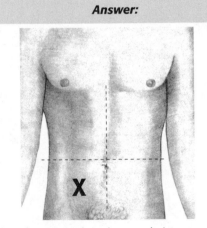

Rationale: Pain and tenderness during an acute attack of appendicitis localize in the right lower quadrant, midway between the umbilicus and the crest of the ilium.

Nursing process step: Data collection

Client needs category: Physiological integrity

Client needs subcategory: Physiological adaptation

Cognitive level: Knowledge

12. A client is admitted to the hospital for routine outpatient surgery. Before surgery, the nurse auscultates the client's chest for breath sounds. Identify the area where the nurse should expect to hear bronchovesicular breath sounds.

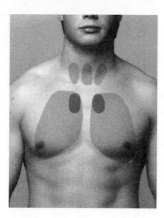

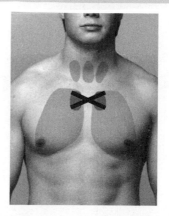

Rationale: Bronchovesicular breath sounds are best heard next to the upper third of the sternum and between the scapulae. These breath sounds are equal in length during inspiration and expiration.

Nursing process step: Data collection

Client needs category: Health promotion and maintenance

Client needs subcategory: None

Cognitive level: Knowledge

PART TWO

Medical-surgical nursing

Cardiovascular disorders

1. A client with a history of hypertension has just had a total hip replacement. The physician orders hydrochlorothiazide (Hydro-Chlor) 35 mg oral solution by mouth, once per day. The label on the solution reads hydrochlorothiazide 50 mg/5 ml. To administer the correct dose, how many ml should the nurse pour?

_____

Answer: 3.5

Rationale: The correct formula to calculate a drug dosage is:

Dose on hand/Quantity on hand = Dose desired/X.

In this example, the equation is:

$$50 \text{ mg}/5 \text{ ml} = 35 \text{ mg}/X$$

$$X = 3.5 \text{ ml.}$$

Nursing process step: Implementation

Client needs category: Physiological integrity

Client needs subcategory: Pharmacological therapies

Cognitive level: Application

2. A client on telemetry reports that she's having chest pain. The hospital unit has standing orders that allow a nurse to begin treating the client before notifying the physician. Place the following actions in proper ascending chronological order. Use all the options.

1. Evaluate the client's response.
2. Administer SL nitroglycerin.
3. Administer oxygen at 2 L/min.
4. Check vital signs.

Answer:

3. Administer oxygen at 2 L/min.
4. Check vital signs.
2. Administer SL nitroglycerin.
1. Evaluate the client's response.

Rationale: Oxygen at 2 to 4 L/min via nasal cannula is a first-line agent to treat myocardial oxygen deficit. Checking vital signs, particularly blood pressure, is important before administering SL nitroglycerin. The nurse will evaluate the effectiveness of the treatment given, document it, and report to the physician.

Nursing process step: Implementation

Client needs category: Physiological integrity

Client needs subcategory: Physiological adaptation

Cognitive level: Analysis

3. A nurse is checking a client who's at risk for cardiac tamponade due to chest trauma sustained in a motorcycle accident. What's the client's pulse pressure if his blood pressure is 108/82 mm Hg?

_____

Rationale: Pulse pressure is the difference between systolic and diastolic pressures. Normally, systolic pressure exceeds diastolic pressure by about 40 mm Hg. Narrowed pulse pressure, a difference of less than 30 mm Hg, is a sign of cardiac tamponade.

Nursing process step: Data collection

Client needs category: Physiological integrity

Client needs subcategory: Physiological adaptation

Cognitive level: Application

---

4. A nurse is preparing to take the blood pressure of a client. Which actions are appropriate? Select all the apply.

☐ **1.** Selecting a cuff that's 80% of arm circumference

☐ **2.** Wrapping the cuff so that the lower border is 8 cm above the antecubital space

☐ **3.** Centering the bladder of the cuff over the brachial artery

☐ **4.** Inflating the cuff to 30 mm above the reading where the brachial pulse disappeared

☐ **5.** Quickly releasing the bulb valve so the pressure drops more than 5 mm Hg per second

Rationale: To obtain an accurate blood pressure reading, the bladder should be 80% of the arm circumference. The nurse should wrap the cuff so that the lower border of the cuff is 2 cm (not 8 cm) above the antecubital space with the bladder centered over the brachial artery. The cuff should be inflated 30 mm Hg above the reading where the brachial pulse disappeared to ensure an accurate assessment of the systolic blood pressure. The bulb valve should be released slowly so pressure drops about 2 to 3 mm Hg per second; inaccurate measurement may occur if the deflation rate is faster.

Nursing process step: Data collection

Client needs category: Physiological integrity

Client needs subcategory: Reduction of risk potential

Cognitive level: Application

5. A nurse is applying a 3-lead telemetry unit to a client newly admitted to the telemetry unit. The client is to be monitored in a lead MCL_1. Identify the area where the nurse would correctly place the positive chest lead.

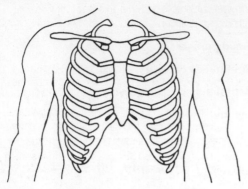

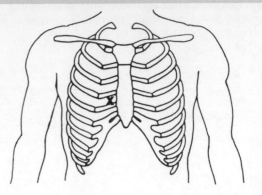

Rationale: Standard placement of the MCL_1 positive chest lead is at the fourth intercostal space to the right of the sternum.

Nursing process: Data collection

Client needs category: Health promotion & maintenance

Client needs subcategory: None

Cognitive level: Application

---

6. A nurse is caring for a client who just underwent cardiac catheterization through a femoral access site. Which nursing interventions should the nurse expect in the care plan for the next 8 hours? Select all that apply.

☐ **1.** Maintain pressure over the femoral access site.

☐ **2.** Allow the client to sit upright for meals.

☐ **3.** Check the dressing and access site for bleeding.

☐ **4.** Monitor vital signs every 4 hours.

☐ **5.** Keep the extremity straight.

☐ **6.** Allow use of the bedside commode.

Answer: 1, 3, 5

Rationale: Pressure should be applied at the access site to control bleeding and promote clot formation. The dressing and access site must be observed frequently for bleeding and hematoma formation. When the femoral access site is used, the head of the bed may not be raised greater than 30 degrees and the affected leg must be kept extended. Therefore, the client may not sit upright for meals or use the bedside commode. Following this procedure, the nurse should monitor vital signs every 15 minutes for the first hour, every 30 minutes for the next 2 hours, and every 4 hours after that.

Nursing process step: Planning

Client needs category: Physiological integrity

Client needs subcategory: Reduction of risk potential

Cognitive level: Application

7. A nurse is assisting with preparing a teaching plan for a client who recently underwent surgery for insertion of a permanent pacemaker. Which instructions should the nurse include in the teaching plan? Select all that apply.

- ☐ **1.** Check heart rate for 1 minute daily.
- ☐ **2.** Check respiratory rate for 1 minute daily.
- ☐ **3.** Report any bulging at the insertion site.
- ☐ **4.** Report redness, swelling, or discharge at the insertion site.
- ☐ **5.** Stay away from airport metal detectors.
- ☐ **6.** Avoid magnetic resonance imaging (MRI) diagnostic studies.

Answer: 1, 4, 6

Rationale: The client with an implanted pacemaker should assess his heart rate daily and report rates that are too fast or too slow. The nurse should instruct him to inspect the insertion site and report signs and symptoms of infection, such as redness, swelling, and discharge. MRI studies are contraindicated in the client with a permanent pacemaker because the magnet may move the metal pacemaker within the body, causing injury. It isn't necessary to obtain a respiratory rate to assess functioning of a pacemaker. A slight bulge at the pacemaker insertion is normal. It's safe for a client with a pacemaker to go through an airport metal detector, but the pacemaker may activate the metal detector. The client should carry his pacemaker identification card to show to security personnel.

Nursing process step: Planning

Client needs category: Physiological integrity

Client needs subcategory: Reduction of risk potential

Cognitive level: Application

---

8. A nurse is assisting in admitting a client with substernal chest pain. Which diagnostic tests does the nurse anticipate the client will receive to confirm or rule out a diagnosis of myocardial infarction (MI)? Select all that apply.

- ☐ **1.** Serum bilirubin
- ☐ **2.** Serum troponin
- ☐ **3.** Serum myoglobin
- ☐ **4.** Urinalysis
- ☐ **5.** Electroencephalogram
- ☐ **6.** 24-hour creatinine clearance

Answer: 2, 3

Rationale: Troponin and myoglobin are enzymes that are released when cardiac muscle is damaged. Serum troponin levels increase within 4 to 6 hours after an MI. Serum myoglobin levels increase within 1 to 3 hours after an MI. Serum bilirubin evaluates liver function and is not altered with cardiac damage. Urinalysis and 24-hour creatinine clearance reflect kidney—not cardiac—function. An electroencephalogram evaluates the electrical activity of the brain.

Nursing process step: Data collection

Client needs category: Physiological integrity

Client needs subcategory: Physiological adaptation

Cognitive level: Application

9. Which signs and symptoms should the nurse expect to find in a client with angina? Select all that apply.

☐ **1.** Chest tightness

☐ **2.** General muscle aching

☐ **3.** Chest pressure

☐ **4.** Jaw pain

☐ **5.** Slowed respiratory rate

☐ **6.** Bradycardia

Rationale: Chest tightness, chest pressure, and jaw pain are all symptoms of angina. General muscle aching is not associated with angina. Respirations and heart rate typically increase, not decrease, with anginal attacks.

Nursing process step: Data collection

Client needs category: Physiological integrity

Client needs subcategory: Physiological adaptation

Cognitive level: Application

---

10. A client is diagnosed with myocardial infarction. Which data collected indicate that the client has developed left-sided heart failure? Select all that apply.

☐ **1.** Ascites

☐ **2.** Jugular vein distention

☐ **3.** Orthopnea

☐ **4.** Cough

☐ **5.** Hepatomegaly

☐ **6.** Crackles

Rationale: Left-sided heart failure produces primarily pulmonary signs and symptoms, such as orthopnea, cough, and crackles. Right-sided heart failure primarily produces systemic signs and symptoms, such as ascites, jugular vein distention, and hepatomegaly.

Nursing process step: Data collection

Client needs category: Physiological integrity

Client needs subcategory: Physiological adaptation

Cognitive level: Application

11. A nurse is performing a cardiac check on a client with hypertension. Identify the area where the nurse should place the stethoscope to best auscultate the pulmonic valve.

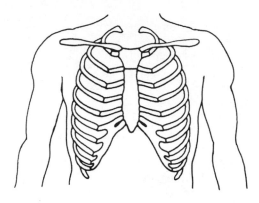

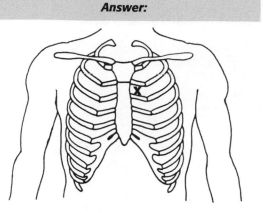

Rationale: Typically, the pulmonic valve is best heard at the second intercostal space, at the left sternal border.

Nursing process step: Data collection

Client needs category: Physiological integrity

Client needs subcategory: Physiological adaptation

Cognitive level: Application

---

12. The nurse is checking the peripheral pulses of a client who underwent cardiac catheterization through the left groin. Identify the area where the nurse should palpate the left posterior tibial artery.

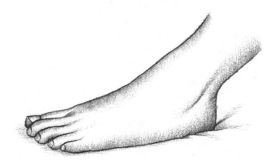

Answer:

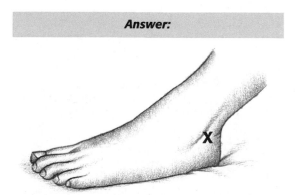

Rationale: The posterior tibial pulse is located behind and just below the lateral malleolus of the foot.

Nursing process step: Data collection

Client needs category: Physiological integrity

Client needs subcategory: Reduction of risk potential

Cognitive level: Knowledge

13. A client with atrial fibrillation is diagnosed with an embolic stroke. Identify the heart chamber that is the most likely source of the fragmented clot responsible for the stroke.

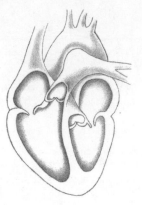

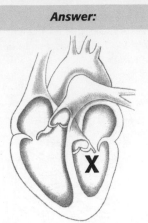

Rationale: Clients with atrial fibrillation are at increased risk for clot formation in the left ventricle of the heart due to stagnation of blood. If a piece of the clot breaks loose and travels to the brain, the client suffers an embolic stroke.

Nursing process step: Data collection

Client needs category: Physiological integrity

Client needs subcategory: Physiological adaptation

Cognitive level: Analysis

Oncologic disorders

1. A client in the terminal stage of cancer is being transferred to hospice care. Which information should the nurse include in the teaching plan regarding hospice care? Select all that apply.

- ☐ **1.** Care focuses on controlling symptoms and relieving pain.
- ☐ **2.** A multidisciplinary team provides care.
- ☐ **3.** Services are based on the client's ability to pay.
- ☐ **4.** Hospice care is provided only in hospice centers.
- ☐ **5.** Bereavement care is provided to the family.
- ☐ **6.** Care is provided in the home independent of physicians.

Answer: 1, 2, 5

Rationale: Hospice care focuses on controlling symptoms and relieving pain at the end of life. Care is provided by a multidisciplinary team that may consist of nurses, physicians, chaplains, aides, and volunteers. After the client's death, hospice provides bereavement care to the grieving family. Hospice care is provided based on need, not on ability to pay. It's provided in various settings, including hospice centers, homes, hospitals, and long-term care facilities. Care is provided under the direction of a physician, who is a key member of the hospice care team.

Nursing process step: Planning

Client needs category: Physiological integrity

Client needs subcategory: Basic care and comfort

Cognitive level: Application

2. A physician has ordered filgrastim (Neupogen) 5 mcg/kg subcutaneously for a postchemotherapy client. The client weighs 140 lb. Neupogen comes in a vial of 300 mcg/ml. How many milliliters of Neupogen will a nurse deliver to the client?

_____

Answer: 1

Rationale: Use the following equation:

$$140 \text{ lb}/2.2 \text{ kg} = 63 \text{ kg}$$

$$63 \text{ kg} \times 5 \text{ mcg} = 315 \text{ mcg/kg}$$

$$300/1 = 315/X$$

$$300X = 315$$

$$X = 1.05 \text{ ml.}$$

Nursing process step: Implementation

Client needs category: Physiological integrity

Client needs subcategory: Pharmacological therapies

Cognitive level: Application

---

3. A nurse is teaching a community program on breast self-examination. She tells the group the proper steps to take when palpating each breast. Place the following actions in proper ascending chronological order. Use all the options.

1. Use the right hand for the left breast (and vice versa).
2. Lie down with your arm behind your head.
3. Palpate the breast in a perpendicular motion going across the breast from side to side and top to bottom.
4. Use a circular motion to feel breast tissue (with light, medium, and firm pressure).
5. Use the finger pads of the three middle fingers.

Answer:

2. Lie down with your arm behind your head.
1. Use the right hand for the left breast (and vice versa).
5. Use the finger pads of the three middle fingers.
4. Use a circular motion to feel breast tissue (with light, medium, and firm pressure).
3. Palpate the breast in a perpendicular motion going across the breast from side to side and top to bottom.

Rationale: Breast self-examination is a standard procedure described by organizations like the American Cancer Society. In addition to the actions listed above, the examination should also include a visual inspection of the breasts while pressing the hands firmly against the hips and an examination of the underarms of each breast with the arms slightly raised.

Nursing process step: Implementation

Client needs category: Health promotion and maintenance

Client needs subcategory: None

Cognitive level: Application

4. A client with breast cancer was admitted earlier in the day with sepsis and complaints of nausea, pain, and lethargy. She completed her third round of chemotherapy last week. A physician has just ordered I.V. D_5 half normal saline solution at 150 ml/hr. Which notes would the nurse expect to see documented in the client's chart? Select all that apply.

☐ **1.** Skin flushed and warm.

☐ **2.** Client groggy but answers questions appropriately.

☐ **3.** Auscultation of lungs: clear bilaterally.

☐ **4.** Abdomen soft and nontender. Bowel sounds present in all quadrants.

☐ **5.** BP 96/50, HR 114/min, RR 22/min, T 103.2°F (39.5°C). Urine output 150 ml in the past 6 hours.

☐ **6.** BUN 35, creatinine 0.4, Na 134, K 4.2, Cl 104.

Answer: 1, 2, 5, 6

Rationale: Due to the infectious process and nausea, alteration in fluid balance is a concern. With the client having flushed warm skin, a groggy mental status, low blood pressure, elevated heart rate and temperature, and deceased urine output, fluid balance becomes more definitive. Elevated BUN level with normal serum creatinine level, and slightly decreased sodium levels with normal potassium levels all confirm dehydration as a significant problem. Therefore, a replacement fluid I.V. would be expected.

Nursing process step: Data collection

Client needs category: Physiological integrity

Client needs subcategory: Physiological adaptation

Cognitive level: Analysis

---

5. A client with laryngeal cancer has undergone laryngectomy and is receiving radiation therapy to the head and neck. The nurse should monitor the client for which adverse effects of external radiation? Select all that apply.

☐ **1.** Xerostomia

☐ **2.** Stomatitis

☐ **3.** Thrombocytopenia

☐ **4.** Cystitis

☐ **5.** Dysgeusia

☐ **6.** Leukopenia

Answer: 1, 2, 5

Rationale: Radiation of the head and neck commonly causes xerostomia (dry mouth), stomatitis (irritation of the oral mucous membranes), and dysgeusia (a diminished sense of taste). Thrombocytopenia (reduced platelet count) and leukopenia (reduced white blood cell count) may occur after systemic radiation. Cystitis may occur after radiation of the genitourinary system.

Nursing process step: Data collection

Client needs category: Physiological integrity

Client needs subcategory: Reduction of risk potential

Cognitive level: Application

6. A client with bladder cancer undergoes surgical removal of the bladder and construction of an ileal conduit. Which data indicate that the client is developing complications? Select all that apply.

☐ **1.** Urine output is greater than 30 ml/hr.

☐ **2.** The stoma appears dusky.

☐ **3.** The stoma protrudes from the skin.

☐ **4.** Mucus shreds are in the urine collection bag.

☐ **5.** Edema of the stoma is present during the first 24 hours postoperatively.

☐ **6.** The client experiences sharp abdominal pain and abdominal rigidity.

Rationale: A dusky appearance of the stoma indicates decreased blood supply; a healthy stoma should appear beefy-red. Protrusion indicates prolapse of the stoma. Sharp abdominal pain and rigidity suggest peritonitis. A urine output greater than 30 ml/hr is a sign of adequate renal perfusion and is a normal finding. Because mucous membranes are used to create the conduit, mucus in the urine is expected. Stomal edema is a normal finding during the first 24 hours after surgery.

Nursing process step: Data collection

Client needs category: Physiological integrity

Client needs subcategory: Reduction of risk potential

Cognitive level: Analysis

---

7. A client receiving chemotherapy for breast cancer develops myelosuppression. Which instructions should the nurse expect in the discharge teaching plan? Select all that apply.

☐ **1.** Avoid people who have recently received attenuated vaccines.

☐ **2.** Avoid activities that may cause bleeding.

☐ **3.** Wash hands frequently.

☐ **4.** Increase intake of fresh fruits and vegetables.

☐ **5.** Avoid crowded places such as shopping malls.

☐ **6.** Treat a sore throat with over-the-counter products.

Rationale: Chemotherapy can cause myelosuppression (reduced numbers of red blood cells, white blood cells, and platelets). Clients receiving chemotherapy need to avoid people who have recently been vaccinated because such interaction may exaggerate myelosuppression. In addition, chemotherapy clients should avoid activities that could cause trauma and bleeding because of their reduced platelet counts. Frequent hand washing is the best way to prevent the spread of infection. They should also avoid crowded places and people with colds during the flu season because of their reduced ability to fight infection. Fresh fruits and vegetables should be avoided because they can harbor bacteria that aren't easily removed by washing. Signs and symptoms of infection such as a sore throat, fever, or cough, should be reported immediately to the physician.

Nursing process step: Planning

Client needs category: Physiological integrity

Client needs subcategory: Reduction of risk potential

Cognitive level: Application

8. A client is ordered a dose of epoetin alfa (Procrit). The recommended dosage is 150 units/kg subcutaneously. The client weighs 60 kg. Epoetin alfa comes in a vial of 10,000 units/ml. How many milliliters of epoetin alfa would the nurse expect to administer?

Answer: 0.9

Rationale: Use the following equation:

$$60 \text{ kg} \times 150 \text{ mg} = 9,000 \text{ mg/kg}$$

$$10,000 \text{ units}/1 \text{ ml} = 9,000 \text{ units}/X$$

$$10,000X = 9,000$$

$$X = 0.9 \text{ ml.}$$

Nursing process step: Implementation

Client needs category: Physiological integrity

Client needs subcategory: Pharmacological therapy

Cognitive level: Application

Gastrointestinal disorders

1. A nurse is caring for a client who can't swallow tablets. The client weighs 56 kg. Famotidine (Pepcid) is ordered; it's dispensed as an oral suspension of 40 mg/5 ml. The order states to give Pepcid 0.7 mg/kg/day divided twice daily. How many milliliters would the nurse pour into the medication cup for the first dose?

Answer: 2.5

Rationale: 0.7 mg/kg/day divided twice daily is:

$$0.7 \text{ mg/kg} \times 56 \text{ kg} = 39.2 \text{ mg daily}$$

$$39.2 \text{ mg} \div 2 \text{ doses} = 19.6 \text{ mg; round up to } 20 \text{ mg/dose.}$$

Now use the ratio method to determine the number of milliliters:

$$40 \text{ mg/5 ml} = 20\text{mg}/X \text{ ml}$$

$$40X = 100$$

$$X = 2.5 \text{ ml.}$$

Nursing process step: Implementation

Client needs category: Physiological integrity

Client needs subcategory: Pharmacological therapies

Cognitive level: Application

2. A nurse is teaching a client with an ostomy how to apply a new appliance. Place the nurse's instructions in ascending chronological order. Use all the options.

1.	Add ¹⁄₁₆ to ¹⁄₈ inch to the size of the stoma.
2.	Wash stoma area and pat dry.
3.	Apply thin layer of paste around stoma.
4.	Cut stoma opening into wafer.
5.	Apply pouch.
6.	Measure the stoma size.

Answer:

2.	Wash stoma area and pat dry.
6.	Measure the stoma size.
1.	Add ¹⁄₁₆ to ¹⁄₈ inch to the size of the stoma.
4.	Cut stoma opening into wafer.
3.	Apply thin layer of paste around stoma.
5.	Apply pouch.

Rationale: Standardized protocols exist for changing an ostomy pouch. Materials for client education are available from a number of national agencies. Adhesive remover is used to promote skin integrity when removing the old pouch. After washing, the skin must be gently but thoroughly dried. Once the stoma size is determined, an area of ¹⁄₁₆ to ¹⁄₈ inch is added so that the stoma is independent of any barrier. A thin layer of paste is used to help maintain the pouch seal. Pouches can remain in place for up to 7 days if the seal is unbroken.

Nursing Process Step: Implementation

Client Needs Category: Health promotion and maintenance

Client Needs Subcategory: None

Cognitive Level: Application

---

3. As part of a routine screening for colorectal cancer, a client must undergo fecal occult blood testing. Which foods should the nurse instruct the client to avoid 48 to 72 hours before the test and throughout the collection period? Select all that apply.

☐ **1.** High-fiber foods

☐ **2.** Red meat

☐ **3.** Turnips

☐ **4.** Cantaloupe

☐ **5.** Tomatoes

☐ **6.** Peas

Answer: 2, 3, 4

Rationale: The client should be instructed to maintain a high-fiber diet and to refrain from eating red meat, poultry, fish, turnips, and cantaloupe for 48 to 72 hours before the test and throughout the collection period. High-fiber diets help to increase stool volume and decrease colonic transit time and intraluminal pressure, thus preventing constipation.

Nursing process step: Implementation

Client needs category: Health promotion and maintenance

Client needs subcategory: None

Cognitive level: Application

4. A client with osteoarthritis is admitted to the hospital with peptic ulcer disease. Which findings are commonly associated with peptic ulcer disease? Select all that apply.

☐ **1.** Localized, colicky periumbilical pain

☐ **2.** History of nonsteroidal anti-inflammatory use

☐ **3.** Epigastric pain that's relieved by antacids

☐ **4.** Tachycardia

☐ **5.** Nausea and weight loss

☐ **6.** Low-grade fever

Rationale: Peptic ulcer disease is characterized by nausea, hematemesis, melena, weight loss, and left-sided epigastric pain that occurs 1 to 2 hours after eating and is relieved with antacids. Nonsteroidal anti-inflammatory drug use is also associated with peptic ulcer disease. Appendicitis begins with generalized or localized colicky periumbilical or epigastric pain, followed by anorexia, nausea, a few episodes of vomiting, low-grade fever, and tachycardia.

Nursing process step: Data collection

Client needs category: Physiological integrity

Client needs subcategory: Physiological adaptation

Cognitive level: Analysis

---

5. A client undergoes a barium swallow fluoroscopy that confirms gastroesophageal reflux disease (GERD). Based on this diagnosis, the client should be instructed to take which actions? Select all that apply.

☐ **1.** Follow a high-fat, low-fiber diet.

☐ **2.** Avoid caffeine and carbonated beverages.

☐ **3.** Sleep with the head of the bed flat.

☐ **4.** Stop smoking.

☐ **5.** Take antacids 1 hour and 3 hours after meals.

☐ **6.** Limit alcohol consumption to one drink per day.

Answer: 2, 4, 5

Rationale: The nurse should instruct the client with GERD to follow a low-fat, high-fiber diet. Caffeine, carbonated beverages, alcohol, and smoking should be avoided because they aggravate GERD. In addition, the client should take antacids as prescribed (typically 1 hour and 3 hours after meals and at bedtime). Lying down with the head of the bed elevated, not flat, reduces intra-abdominal pressure, thereby reducing the symptoms of GERD.

Nursing process step: Implementation

Client needs category: Health promotion and maintenance

Client needs subcategory: None

Cognitive level: Application

6. A client with constipation is prescribed an irrigating enema. Which steps should the nurse take when administering an enema? Select all that apply.

☐ **1.** Assist the client into the left-lateral Sims' position.

☐ **2.** Lubricate the distal end of the rectal catheter.

☐ **3.** Warm the solution to 110° F (43.3° C).

☐ **4.** Insert the tube 1″ to 1½″.

☐ **5.** Administer 250 to 500 ml of irrigating solution.

☐ **6.** Be sure to keep the solution container no higher than 18″ above bed level.

Answer: 1, 2, 6

Rationale: To administer an enema, the nurse should prepare the prescribed type and amount of solution. The standard volume of an irrigating enema for an adult is 750 to 1,000 ml. For an adult, the solution should be warmed to 100° (37.8° C) to 105° F (40.6° C) to help reduce client discomfort. The nurse should help the client into the left-lateral Sims' position. After lubricating the distal end of the rectal catheter, the nurse should insert the tube 2″ to 3″. During infusion, the solution bag shouldn't be raised higher than 18″ above bed level.

Nursing process step: Implementation

Client needs category: Physiological integrity

Client needs subcategory: Basic care and comfort

Cognitive level: Application

---

7. A client with cirrhosis is ordered to have a daily measurement of his abdominal girth. Identify the anatomic landmark where the tape measure should be placed when obtaining this measurement.

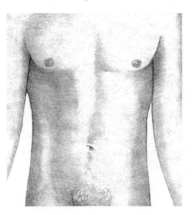

Answer:

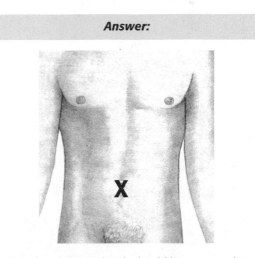

Rationale: Abdominal girth should be measured at the umbilicus to obtain the most accurate measurement. Using any other anatomic landmark wouldn't provide the correct measurement for the client's abdominal girth.

Nursing process step: Data collection

Client needs category: Health promotion and maintenance

Client needs subcategory: None

Cognitive level: Application

8. A client undergoes colonoscopy for colorectal cancer screening. A polyp was removed during the procedure. Which nursing interventions are necessary when caring for the client immediately after colonoscopy? Select all that apply.

- ☐ **1.** When the client recovers from sedation, tell him he must follow a clear liquid diet.
- ☐ **2.** Instruct the client that he shouldn't drive for 24 hours.
- ☐ **3.** Observe the client closely for signs and symptoms of bowel perforation.
- ☐ **4.** Monitor vital signs frequently until they're stable.
- ☐ **5.** Inform the client that there may be blood in his stool and that he should report excessive blood immediately.
- ☐ **6.** Tell the client to report excessive flatus.

Answer: 3, 4, 5

Rationale: After colonoscopy, the nurse should observe the client closely for signs and symptoms of bowel perforation (malaise, rectal bleeding, abdominal pain and distention, fever, and mucopurulent drainage). The nurse should monitor vital signs frequently until they become stable. Because a polyp was removed during the procedure, the nurse should inform the client that there may be some blood in his stool and that he should report excessive bleeding immediately. The nurse should tell the client he might pass large amounts of flatus resulting from air insufflated to distend the colon but it's not necessary to report it. When the client has recovered from sedation, he may resume his usual diet; a clear liquid diet isn't necessary. The client shouldn't drive for 12 hours after being sedated.

Nursing process step: Implementation

Client needs category: Health promotion and maintenance

Client needs subcategory: None

Cognitive level: Application

---

9. A client has been hospitalized with pancreatitis for 3 days. A nurse checks the client and documents the results below. The nurse realizes that this information is a manifestation of what finding?

6/28/06 1415	Skin warm and dry. Color pink with no signs of pallor. BP 156/84, HR 102/min, RR 22/min. O_2 at 2 L/min via nasal cannula. O_2 saturation 98%. Denies any shortness of breath. Bowel sounds present in all four quadrants. Patient states he has pain-rated at 8 on pain scale of 0-10. NG tube to low intermittent suction— light green drainage present. NG tube placement verified; pH of 3. Periumbilical area appears discolored and ecchymotic. ————————F. Johnson, LPN

- ☐ **1.** Cullen's sign
- ☐ **2.** Chvostek's sign
- ☐ **3.** Trousseau's sign
- ☐ **4.** Broca's sign

Answer: 1

Rationale: Cullen's sign is a discoloration at the periumbilical area. Its presence may indicate an underlying subcutaneous intraperitoneal hemorrhage. Chvostek's sign is a facial nerve spasm and Trousseau's sign is a carpopedal spasm, both in response to hypocalcemia. Broca's area is located within the brain.

Nursing Process Step: Data collection

Client Needs Category: Physiological integrity

Client Needs Subcategory: Physiologic adaptation

Cognitive Level: Analysis

10. A client with a retroperitoneal abscess is receiving gentamicin (Garamycin) I.V. Which levels should the nurse monitor? Select all that apply.

☐ **1.** Hearing

☐ **2.** Urine output

☐ **3.** Hematocrit (HCT)

☐ **4.** Blood urea nitrogen (BUN) and creatinine

☐ **5.** Serum calcium

Answer: 1, 2, 4

Rationale: Adverse reactions to gentamicin include ototoxicity and nephrotoxicity. The nurse must monitor the client's hearing and instruct him to report any hearing loss or tinnitus. Signs of nephrotoxicity include decreased urine output and elevated BUN and creatinine levels. Gentamicin doesn't affect HCT or serum calcium level.

Nursing process step: Data collection

Client needs category: Physiological integrity

Client needs subcategory: Pharmacological therapies

Cognitive level: Analysis

---

11. Locate the abdominal quadrant where the nurse would expect to palpate the liver.

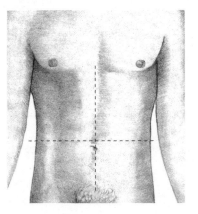

Answer:

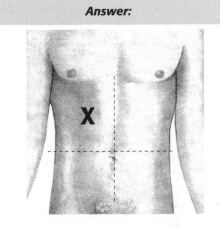

Rationale: The liver is located in the right upper abdominal quadrant.

Nursing process step: Data collection

Client needs category: Health promotion and maintenance

Client needs subcategory: None

Cognitive level: Knowledge

Integumentary disorders

1. At an outpatient clinic, a medical assistant interviews a client and documents the findings in the chart below. After reading the chart note, a nurse begins planning based on which nursing diagnoses?

12/13/06	Client very anxious because of new black
0900	mole with shades of brown noted on upper
	outer right thigh. Asymmetrical in shape with
	an irregular border. —— M. Rosenfeld, MA

☐ **1.** *Deficient knowledge related to potential diagnosis of basal cell carcinoma*

☐ **2.** *Fear related to potential diagnosis of malignant melanoma*

☐ **3.** *Risk for impaired skin integrity related to potential squamous cell carcinoma*

☐ **4.** *Readiness for enhanced knowledge of skin care precautions related to benign mole*

Answer: 2

Rationale: Documentation reveals the client to be anxious about her symptoms. These signs and symptoms most closely resemble malignant melanoma, due to the asymmetry, variable color, and border irregularity. Thus, *Fear related to potential diagnosis of malignant melanoma* is the most likely nursing diagnosis. The client doesn't express deficient knowledge or readiness for enhanced knowledge presently. The lesion described doesn't resemble basal or squamous cell carcinoma, nor a benign mole.

Nursing process step: Planning

Client needs category: Physiological integrity

Client needs subcategory: Physiological adaptation

Cognitive level: Analysis

---

2. Despite conventional treatment, a client's psoriasis has worsened. The physician prescribes methotrexate 25 mg by mouth as a single weekly dose. The pharmacy dispenses 2.5-mg scored tablets. How many tablets should the nurse instruct the client to consume to achieve the prescribed dose?

_____

Answer: 10

Rationale: The correct formula to calculate a drug dose is:

Dose on hand/Quantity on hand = Dose desired/X.

The physician prescribes 25 mg, which is the dose desired. The pharmacy dispenses 2.5-mg tablets, which is the dose on hand. Therefore:

$$2.5 \text{ mg}/1 \text{ tablet} = 25 \text{ mg}/X \text{ tablets}$$

$$X = 10 \text{ tablets}.$$

Nursing process step: Planning

Client needs category: Physiological integrity

Client needs subcategory: Pharmacological therapies

Cognitive level: Application

3. Which nursing interventions are effective in preventing pressure ulcers? Select all that apply.

☐ **1.** Clean the skin with warm water and a mild cleaning agent; then apply a moisturizer.

☐ **2.** When turning the client, slide him and avoid lifting him.

☐ **3.** Avoid raising the head of the bed more than 90 degrees.

☐ **4.** Turn and reposition the client every 1 to 2 hours unless contraindicated.

☐ **5.** If the client uses a wheelchair, seat him on a rubber or plastic doughnut.

☐ **6.** Use pillows to position the client and increase his comfort.

Answer: 1, 4, 6

Rationale: Nursing interventions that are effective in preventing pressure ulcers include cleaning the skin with warm water and a mild cleaning agent, and then applying a moisturizer; lifting—rather than sliding—the client when turning him to reduce friction and shear; avoiding raising the head of the bed more than 30 degrees, except for brief periods; repositioning and turning the client every 1 to 2 hours unless contraindicated; and using pillows to position the client and increase his comfort. If the client uses a wheelchair, the nurse should offer a pressure-relieving cushion as appropriate. She should not seat him on a rubber or plastic doughnut because these devices can increase localized pressure at vulnerable points.

Nursing process step: Implementation

Client needs category: Safe, effective care environment

Client needs subcategory: Safety and infection control

Cognitive level: Application

---

4. A client has been hospitalized with bacterial pneumonia and dehydration for 3 days. The client's right heel reveals a shallow opened area draining clear fluid, which appears to be a skin tear. The nurse would understand which items related to this client's skin break? Select all that apply.

☐ **1.** The heel wound would be classified as a stage 1 pressure ulcer.

☐ **2.** Increasing fluid intake would help prevent further skin injury.

☐ **3.** The wound is at risk for infection.

☐ **4.** Placing the client on an air mattress will heal the wound.

☐ **5.** The client's caloric requirements are lower than normal because of decreased activity.

☐ **6.** The injured area would be painful to the client.

Answer: 2, 3, 6

Rationale: Good hydration leads to healthier skin that's less prone to injury. This wound is open, which puts it at risk for infection, particularly in a client who already has an underlying infection. Stage 1 and 2 pressure ulcers are generally painful to clients with normal sensation. As nerve cells are destroyed by the pressure and ulceration, wounds become less painful but more serious. Pressure wounds are categorized into four stages, and the client's wound would be considered a stage 2 because the area is open but shallow, and draining serous-type fluid. An air mattress alone will be insufficient; in order for the affected area to heal, direct pressure on the wound must be removed by frequent repositioning. The client's caloric needs have increased due to the need to grow new tissue and recover from a lung infection.

Nursing Process Step: Data collection

Client Needs Category: Physiological integrity

Client Needs Subcategory: Physiological adaptation

Cognitive Level: Application

---

5. Which instructions should be included in the teaching plan of a client with acne vulgaris who's prescribed tretinoin, benzoyl peroxide, and tetracycline? Select all that apply.

☐ **1.** Expect your skin to look red and start to peel after treatment.

☐ **2.** Take tetracycline on an empty stomach.

☐ **3.** Use tretinoin and benzoyl peroxide together in the morning and at bedtime.

☐ **4.** Maintain the prescribed treatment because it's more likely to improve acne than a strict diet and frequent scrubbing with soap and water.

☐ **5.** Apply tretinoin at least 30 minutes after washing the face and at bedtime.

☐ **6.** Avoid exposure to sunlight and don't use a sunscreen.

Answer: 2, 4

Rationale: The client should be instructed to take tetracycline on an empty stomach. The nurse should also make sure that the client understands that the prescribed treatment is more likely to improve acne than are a strict diet and frequent scrubbing with soap and water. The nurse should instruct the client receiving tretinoin that his skin should look pink and dry after treatment. If the skin appears red or starts to peel, the preparation may have to be weakened or applied less often. Because the prescribed regimen includes tretinoin and benzoyl peroxide, the nurse should instruct the client to use one preparation in the morning and the other at night. Tretinoin should be applied 30 minutes after washing the face and at least 1 hour before bedtime. The nurse should advise the client to avoid exposure to sunlight or to use a sunscreen.

Nursing process step: Planning

Client needs category: Physiological integrity

Client needs subcategory: Pharmacological therapies

Cognitive level: Application

---

6. A client is brought to the emergency department with partial- and full-thickness burns over 15% of his body. His admission vital signs are: blood pressure 100/50 mm Hg, heart rate 130 beats/minute, and respiratory rate 26 breaths/minute. Which nursing interventions are appropriate for this client? Select all that apply.

☐ **1.** Clean the burns with hydrogen peroxide.

☐ **2.** Cover the burns with saline-soaked towels.

☐ **3.** Begin an I.V. infusion of lactated Ringer's solution.

☐ **4.** Place ice directly on the burn areas.

☐ **5.** Administer 6 mg of morphine I.V.

☐ **6.** Administer tetanus prophylaxis, as ordered.

Answer: 3, 5, 6

Rationale: Immediate interventions for this client should aim to stop the burning and relieve the pain. The nurse should begin I.V. therapy with a crystalloid such as lactated Ringer's solution to prevent hypovolemic shock and to maintain cardiac output. She should administer pain medication, as ordered. Typically, 2 to 25 mg of morphine or 5 to 15 mg of meperidine (Demerol) is administered I.V. in small increments. Tetanus prophylaxis should be administered, as ordered. The nurse shouldn't use hydrogen peroxide or povidone-iodine solution to clean the burns because these preparations can further damage tissue. The nurse should avoid the use of saline-soaked towels because they may lead to hypothermia. Ice should not be placed directly on burn wounds because the cold may cause further thermal damage.

Nursing process step: Implementation

Client needs category: Physiological integrity

Client needs subcategory: Physiological adaptation

Cognitive level: Application

Immune and hematologic disorders

1. A nurse is assisting in planning care for a client with human immunodeficiency virus (HIV). Which statements by the nurse indicate an understanding of HIV transmission? Select all that apply.

☐ **1.** "I will wear a gown, mask, and gloves with all client contact."

☐ **2.** "I don't need to wear any personal protective equipment due to decreased risk of occupational exposure."

☐ **3.** "I will wear a mask if the client has a cough caused by an upper respiratory infection."

☐ **4.** "I will wear a mask, gown, and gloves when splashing of bodily fluids is likely."

☐ **5.** "I will wash my hands after client care."

Answer: 4, 5

Rationale: Standard precautions include wearing gloves for any known or anticipated contact with blood, body fluids, tissue, mucous membranes, and nonintact skin. If the task or procedure may result in splashing or splattering of blood or body fluids to the face, the nurse should wear a mask and goggles or face shield. If the task or procedure may result in splashing or splattering of blood or body fluids, the nurse should wear a fluid-resistant gown or apron. Hands should be washed before and after client care and after removing gloves. A gown, mask, and gloves aren't necessary for all client care unless contact with bodily fluids, tissue, mucous membranes, and nonintact skin is expected. Nurses have an increased, not decreased, risk of occupational exposure to bloodborne pathogens. HIV is not transmitted in sputum unless blood is present.

Nursing process step: Planning

Client needs category: Safe, effective care environment

Client needs subcategory: Safety and infection control

Cognitive level: Application

2. A client is having an anaphylactic reaction. The code team is present and the physician orders epinephrine 1:1000 aqueous solution 0.5 mg subcutaneously stat. A nurse has a prefilled syringe of 1:1000 1 mg/ml epinephrine. The nurse will administer how many milliliters of epinephrine?

_____

Answer: 0.5

Rationale: Use the following equation:

$$1/1 = 0.5/X$$

$$1X = 0.5$$

$$X = 0.5 \text{ ml.}$$

Nursing process step: Implementation

Client needs category: Physiological integrity

Client needs subcategory: Pharmacological therapy

Cognitive level: Application

3. A client is admitted with an exacerbation of Crohn's disease and has a history of lupus erythematosus. A maculopapular rash is present over the client's nose and cheeks. The client denies that the rash itches or is painful. The nurse concludes which of the following? Select all that apply.

☐ **1.** The client is overheated and the rash will disappear once it's bathed in cool water.

☐ **2.** The rash is normal and doesn't need to be addressed.

☐ **3.** The physician must be notified of the rash immediately.

☐ **4.** The rash is a consequence of the corticosteroids (that must now be changed) originally ordered to treat Crohn's disease.

☐ **5.** The rash is a result of poor hygiene and will resolve with proper cleansing.

☐ **6.** Contact precautions will need to be ordered for this client's care.

Answer: 2

Rationale: A butterfly rash on the face may be seen in systemic lupus erythematosus and may be characterized by a malar erythema to discoid lesions. Notifying the physician is not warranted. The rash does not appear as a result of medication, nor is it a result of environmental factors such as heat or hygiene. Considering the rash is related to lupus and isn't contagious, contact precautions aren't necessary.

Nursing process step: Data collection

Client needs category: Health promotion and maintenance

Client needs subcategory: None

Cognitive level: Application

---

4. A nurse is preparing a client with systemic lupus erythematosus (SLE) for discharge. Which instructions should the nurse expect in the teaching plan? Select all that apply.

☐ **1.** Stay out of direct sunlight.

☐ **2.** Refrain from limiting activity between flare-ups.

☐ **3.** Monitor body temperature.

☐ **4.** Taper the corticosteroid dosage as ordered by the physician, when symptoms are under control.

☐ **5.** Apply cold packs to relieve joint pain and stiffness.

Answer: 1, 3, 4

Rationale: The client with SLE should stay out of direct sunlight and avoid other sources of ultraviolet light because they may precipitate severe skin reactions and exacerbate the disease. The client should monitor his temperature because fever can signal an exacerbation, which should be reported to the physician. Corticosteroids must be tapered gradually once symptoms are relieved because they can suppress the function of the adrenal glands. Stopping corticosteroids abruptly can cause adrenal insufficiency, a potentially life-threatening condition. Fatigue can cause a flare-up of SLE; encourage clients to pace activities and plan for rest periods. The client should apply heat, not cold, to relieve joint pain. Cold packs may aggravate Raynaud's phenomenon, which commonly occurs in clients with SLE.

Nursing process step: Planning

Client needs category: Physiological integrity

Client needs subcategory: Reduction of risk potential

Cognitive level: Application

5. A nurse is preparing a client for bone marrow biopsy to rule out leukemia. The nurse explains that the sample will be taken from the anterior iliac crest. Identify this area.

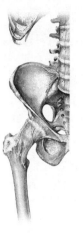

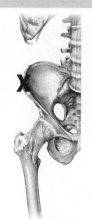

Rationale: A bone marrow biopsy may be taken from the anterior or posterior iliac crests, sternum, vertebral spinous process, rib, or tibia.

Nursing process step: Implementation

Client needs category: Physiological integrity

Client needs subcategory: Physiological adaptation

Cognitive level: Comprehension

---

6. A client with leukemia has enlarged lymph nodes, liver, and spleen. Identify the quadrant of the abdomen where the nurse would find the enlarged spleen.

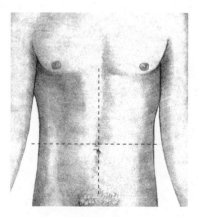

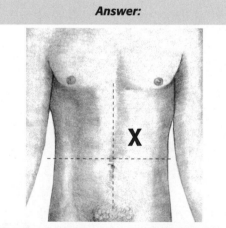

Rationale: The spleen is located in the left upper quadrant of the abdomen, posterior to the stomach.

Nursing process step: Data collection

Client needs category: Physiological integrity

Client needs subcategory: Physiological adaptation

Cognitive level: Comprehension

Endocrine and metabolic disorders

1. A nurse is obtaining information on a newly admitted client who has been diagnosed with diabetes insipidus. Which data should the nurse expect to collect? Select all that apply.

- ☐ **1.** Extreme polyuria
- ☐ **2.** Excessive thirst
- ☐ **3.** Elevated systolic blood pressure
- ☐ **4.** Low urine specific gravity
- ☐ **5.** Bradycardia
- ☐ **6.** Elevated serum potassium level

Answer: 1, 2, 4

Rationale: Signs and symptoms of diabetes insipidus include an abrupt onset of extreme polyuria, excessive thirst, dry skin and mucous membranes, tachycardia, and hypotension. Diagnostic studies reveal low urine specific gravity and osmolarity and elevated serum sodium level. Serum potassium level is likely to be decreased, not increased.

Nursing process: Data collection

Client needs category: Physiological integrity

Client needs subcategory: Physiological adaptation

Cognitive level: Application

---

2. A client has vision problems, so his daughter draws up insulin for him on a weekly basis. The client uses U-100 insulin at 10 units/1 ml, 10 ml/vial. If the client's morning dose of NPH insulin is 5 units, how many syringes can he use before he needs another vial of insulin?

_____

Answer: 20

Rationale: This is a two-step process. First, determine how many milliliters are used in each syringe. There are 10 units/1 ml and the client uses 5 units daily.

$$10 \text{ units/ml} = 5 \text{ units}/X$$

$$0.5 \text{ ml} = X.$$

Second, there's a total of 10 ml in the vial. Determine how many syringes can be filled for doses of 0.5 ml:

$$10 \text{ ml/vial} = 0.5 \text{ ml}/X$$

$$X = 20 \text{ syringes}.$$

Nursing process step: Implementation

Client needs category: Physiological integrity

Client needs subcategory: Pharmacological therapies

Cognitive level: Application

3. A client is on NPH 12 units and Humalog 6 units each morning. Place the following actions in ascending chronological order of how a nurse would demonstrate how to mix insulins. Use all the options.

1.	Withdraw 12 units of NPH insulin.

2.	Inject 12 units of air into NPH vial.

3.	Inject 6 units of air into Humalog vial.

4.	Wipe off vials with alcohol swab.

5.	Withdraw 6 units of Humalog insulin.

Answer:

4.	Wipe off vials with alcohol swab.

2.	Inject 12 units of air into NPH vial.

3.	Inject 6 units of air into Humalog vial.

5.	Withdraw 6 units of Humalog insulin.

1.	Withdraw 12 units of NPH insulin.

Rationale: The insulin bottles should be cleaned of contaminants before each use. Air is injected into the NPH vial first, without touching the insulin. Then, the proper amount of air is inserted into the fast-acting insulin and drawn up into the syringe. Fast- or rapid-acting insulin is drawn into the syringe first to avoid the risk of mixing the long-acting insulin into the vial and delaying the onset of action of the regular insulin in an emergency. Intermediate- or long-acting insulin is drawn into the syringe last. Insulin glargine (Lantus) should never be mixed with another insulin because a precipitate will form and inactivate the drug.

Nursing process step: Implementation

Client needs category: Health promotion and maintenance

Client needs subcategory: None

Cognitive level: Application

---

4. After falling off a ladder and suffering a brain injury, a client develops syndrome of inappropriate antidiuretic hormone (SIADH) secretion. Which of the following findings indicate the effectiveness of the treatment he's receiving? Select all that apply.

☐ **1.** Decrease in body weight

☐ **2.** Rise in blood pressure and drop in heart rate

☐ **3.** Absence of wheezes in the lungs

☐ **4.** Increased urine output

☐ **5.** Decreased urine osmolarity
concentration

Answer: 1, 4, 5

Rationale: SIADH secretion is an abnormality in which there is an abundance of the antidiuretic hormone. The predominant feature is water retention, as well as oliguria, edema, and weight gain. Evidence of successful treatment includes a reduction in weight, an increase in urine output, and a decrease in the urine's concentration (urine osmolarity). Changes in blood pressure, heart rate, and breath sounds aren't characteristic of the disease process.

Nursing process step: Evaluation

Client needs category: Physiological integrity

Client needs subcategory: Physiological adaptation

Cognitive level: Analysis

5. A 48-year-old female client is seen in the clinic for newly diagnosed hypothyroidism. Which topics should the nurse include in a client teaching plan? Select all that apply.

☐ **1.** High-protein, high-calorie diet

☐ **2.** High-fiber, low-calorie diet

☐ **3.** Plan for a thyroidectomy

☐ **4.** Use of stool softeners

☐ **5.** Thyroid hormone replacements

☐ **6.** Review of the procedure for thyroid radiation therapy

Rationale: The treatment for hypothyroidism includes a high-fiber, low-calorie diet because weight gain and constipation are two symptoms of the disorder. Stool softeners are prescribed to prevent constipation, and thyroid hormone replacements are needed to supplement the underfunctioning thyroid gland. A high-protein, high-calorie diet is commonly used for clients with hyperthyroidism, along with thyroidectomy or irradiation of the thyroid gland.

Nursing process step: Planning

Client needs category: Physiological integrity

Client needs subcategory: Reduction of risk potential

Cognitive level: Application

---

6. A client who has been seen in the clinic is scheduled for an outpatient thyroid scan in 2 weeks. Which instructions should the nurse expect in the client teaching points so that this client is prepared? Select all that apply.

☐ **1.** Stop using iodized salt or iodized salt substitutes 1 week before the scan.

☐ **2.** Stop eating seafood 1 week before the scan.

☐ **3.** Don't consume any food or fluids after midnight on the night before the scan.

☐ **4.** Don't take prescribed thyroid medication on the day of the scan.

☐ **5.** Don't take prescribed thyroid medication until the results of the scan are known.

☐ **6.** Maintain bed rest for 24 hours after the scan.

Answer: 1, 2, 4

Rationale: A thyroid scan visualizes the distribution of radioactive dye in the thyroid gland. Interventions before the scan include stopping the ingestion of iodine, which is found in iodized salt, salt substitutes, and seafood. The client should also be instructed not to take any medication that would interfere with the scan. The client doesn't have to refrain from consuming food or fluids after midnight if the scan is done on an outpatient basis. The radioactive dye is administered intravenously. Routinely prescribed medications can be taken after the scan. Bed rest is maintained with a thyroid biopsy, not a scan.

Nursing process step: Implementation

Client needs category: Physiological integrity

Client needs subcategory: Reduction of risk potential

Cognitive level: Application

7. A client is admitted to the hospital with signs and symptoms of diabetes mellitus. Which findings is the nurse most likely to observe in this client? Select all that apply.

☐ **1.** Excessive thirst

☐ **2.** Weight gain

☐ **3.** Constipation

☐ **4.** Excessive hunger

☐ **5.** Urine retention

☐ **6.** Frequent, high-volume urination

Rationale: Classic signs of diabetes mellitus include polydipsia (excessive thirst), polyphagia (excessive hunger), and polyuria (excessive urination). Because the body is starving from the lack of glucose the cells are using for energy, the client has weight loss, not weight gain. Clients with diabetes mellitus usually don't present with constipation. Urine retention is only a problem if the patient has another renal-related condition.

Nursing process step: Data collection

Client needs category: Health promotion and maintenance

Client needs subcategory: None

Cognitive level: Analysis

8. A client is being discharged after having a thyroidectomy. Which discharge instructions are appropriate for this client? Select all that apply.

☐ **1.** Report any signs and symptoms of hypoglycemia.

☐ **2.** Take thyroid replacement medication, as ordered.

☐ **3.** Watch for lethargy, restlessness, sensitivity to cold, and dry skin. Report them to the physician.

☐ **4.** Avoid over-the-counter medications.

☐ **5.** Carry injectable dexamethasone at all times.

Rationale: After removal of the thyroid gland, the client needs to take thyroid replacement medication. The client needs to report to the physician changes in body functioning, such as lethargy, restlessness, cold sensitivity, and dry skin, because they may indicate the need to increase the medication dosage. The thyroid gland doesn't regulate the serum glucose level; therefore, the client wouldn't need to recognize the signs and symptoms of hypoglycemia. A client with Addison's disease should avoid over-the-counter medications and carry injectable dexamethasone.

Nursing process step: Implementation

Client needs category: Physiological integrity

Client needs subcategory: Physiological adaptation

Cognitive level: Application

9. A client is seen in the clinic with suspected parathormone (PTH) deficiency. Part of the diagnosis of this condition includes the analysis of serum electrolyte levels. The levels of which electrolytes would the nurse expect to be abnormal in a client with PTH deficiency? Select all that apply.

- ☐ **1.** Sodium
- ☐ **2.** Potassium
- ☐ **3.** Calcium
- ☐ **4.** Chloride
- ☐ **5.** Glucose
- ☐ **6.** Phosphorus

Answer: 3, 6

Rationale: A client with PTH deficiency has decreased serum calcium and increased phosphorus levels because PTH regulates these two electrolytes. PTH deficiency doesn't affect sodium, potassium, chloride, or glucose levels.

Nursing process step: Evaluation

Client needs category: Health promotion and maintenance

Client needs subcategory: None

Cognitive level: Analysis

---

10. A client is placed on hypocalcemia precautions after removal of the parathyroid gland as a result of cancer. The nurse should observe the client for which symptoms? Select all that apply.

- ☐ **1.** Numbness
- ☐ **2.** Aphasia
- ☐ **3.** Tingling
- ☐ **4.** Muscle twitching and spasms
- ☐ **5.** Polyuria
- ☐ **6.** Polydipsia

Answer: 1, 3, 4

Rationale: When the parathyroid gland is removed, the body may not produce enough parathyroid hormone to regulate calcium and phosphorus levels. The symptoms of hypocalcemia include peripheral numbness, tingling, and muscle spasms. Aphasia isn't a symptom of calcium depletion. Polyuria and polydipsia are symptoms of diabetes mellitus.

Nursing process step: Data collection

Client needs category: Physiological integrity

Client needs subcategory: Reduction of risk potential

Cognitive level: Analysis

11. A client is admitted to the hospital with Cushing's syndrome. Which nursing interventions are appropriate for this client? Select all that apply.

☐ **1.** Assess for peripheral edema.

☐ **2.** Stress the need for a high-calorie, high-carbohydrate diet.

☐ **3.** Measure intake and output.

☐ **4.** Encourage oral fluid intake.

☐ **5.** Weigh the client daily.

☐ **6.** Instruct the client to avoid foods high in potassium.

Answer: 1, 3, 5

Rationale: Because weight gain and edema are common symptoms of Cushing's syndrome, appropriate interventions include assessing for peripheral edema, measuring intake and output, and weighing the client daily. A low-calorie, low-carbohydrate, high-protein diet is ordered for a client with this disorder. Fluid restriction is often prescribed as well. Treatment of Cushing's syndrome includes the administration of potassium replacements; therefore, restricting foods high in potassium wouldn't be appropriate.

Nursing process step: Implementation

Client needs category: Physiological integrity

Client needs subcategory: Physiological adaptation

Cognitive level: Application

---

12. A client with type 2 diabetes mellitus needs instruction on proper foot care. Which instructions should the nurse expect to review in client teaching? Select all that apply.

☐ **1.** Be sure to use scissors to trim toenails.

☐ **2.** Wear cotton socks.

☐ **3.** Apply foot powder after bathing.

☐ **4.** Go barefoot only when you know your home environment.

☐ **5.** See a podiatrist regularly to have your feet checked.

☐ **6.** Wear loose-fitting shoes.

Answer: 2, 3, 5

Rationale: Foot care for a client with diabetes mellitus includes keeping the feet dry with the application of foot powder and wearing cotton socks to absorb moisture. The client should have a podiatrist check his feet regularly to detect problems early. To prevent injury to the feet, the client should be instructed not to cut his toenails with scissors, walk barefoot, or wear loose-fitting shoes.

Nursing process step: Implementation

Client needs category: Physiological integrity

Client needs subcategory: Reduction of risk potential

Cognitive level: Application

Musculoskeletal disorders

1. A client is diagnosed with osteoporosis. Which statements should a nurse include when teaching the client about the disease? Select all that apply.

☐ **1.** It's common in females after menopause.

☐ **2.** It's a degenerative disease characterized by a decrease in bone density.

☐ **3.** It's a congenital disease caused by poor dietary intake of milk products.

☐ **4.** It can cause pain and injury.

☐ **5.** Passive range-of-motion (ROM) exercises can promote bone growth.

☐ **6.** Weight-bearing exercise should be avoided.

Answer: 1, 2, 4

Rationale: Osteoporosis is a degenerative metabolic bone disorder in which the rate of bone resorption accelerates and the rate of bone formation decelerates, thus decreasing bone density. Postmenopausal women are at increased risk for this disorder because of the loss of estrogen. The decrease in bone density can cause pain and injury. Osteoporosis isn't a congenital disorder; however, low calcium intake does contribute to the disorder. Passive ROM exercises may be performed but they won't promote bone growth. Weight-bearing exercise is encouraged because it promotes bone growth.

Nursing process step: Implementation

Client needs category: Physiological integrity

Client needs subcategory: Physiological adaptation

Cognitive level: Application

2. A client is preparing for discharge from the hospital after undergoing an above-the-knee amputation. Which instructions should the nurse expect in the teaching plan for this client? Select all that apply.

☐ **1.** Massage the residual limb away from the suture line.

☐ **2.** Avoid using heat application to ease pain.

☐ **3.** Report twitching, spasms, or phantom limb pain immediately.

☐ **4.** Avoid exposing the skin around the residual limb to excessive perspiration.

☐ **5.** Be sure to perform the prescribed exercises.

☐ **6.** Rub the residual limb with a dry washcloth for 4 minutes three times per day if it is sensitive to touch.

Answer: 4, 5, 6

Rationale: The nurse should advise the client to avoid exposing the skin around the residual limb to excessive perspiration, which can be irritating. She should tell him to perform prescribed exercises to help minimize complications. The nurse should tell the client that if the residual limb is sensitive to touch, he should rub it with a dry washcloth for 4 minutes three times per day. The nurse should tell the client to massage the residual limb toward — not away from — the suture line to mobilize the scar and to prevent its adherence to bone. The client may experience twitching, spasms, or phantom limb pain while his muscles adjust to the amputation. The nurse should advise the client that he can ease these symptoms with heat, massage, or gentle pressure.

Nursing process step: Planning

Client needs category: Physiological integrity

Client needs subcategory: Reduction of risk potential

Cognitive level: Application

3. A client is scheduled for a laminectomy of L1-L2. The nurse is reviewing the teaching about the procedure with the client. Identify the area that the nurse explains will be involved in this client's surgery.

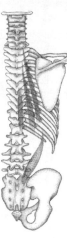

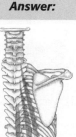

Rationale: In laminectomy, one or more of the bony laminae that cover the vertebrae are removed. There are five lumbar vertebrae, so the nurse can count up from the sacrum to locate L1-L2. Vertebrae are numbered from top to bottom, with L5 being closest to the sacrum.

Nursing process step: Implementation

Client needs category: Physiological integrity

Client needs subcategory: Physiologic adaptation

Cognitive level: Comprehension

---

4. A client is diagnosed with gout. Which foods should the nurse instruct the client to avoid? Select all that apply.

- ☐ **1.** Green leafy vegetables
- ☐ **2.** Liver
- ☐ **3.** Cod
- ☐ **4.** Chocolate
- ☐ **5.** Sardines
- ☐ **6.** Whole milk

Answer: 2, 3, 5

Rationale: The client with gout should avoid foods that are high in purines, such as liver, cod, and sardines. Other foods that should be avoided include anchovies, kidneys, sweetbreads, lentils, and alcoholic beverages, especially beer and wine. Green leafy vegetables, chocolate, and whole milk aren't high in purines and, therefore, aren't restricted in the diet of a client with gout.

Nursing process step: Implementation

Client needs category: Physiological integrity

Client needs subcategory: Basic care and comfort

Cognitive level: Application

5. A client is about to undergo total hip replacement surgery. Before the surgery, the nurse reviews preoperative teaching with him. The nurse can tell that the teaching her been effective when the client verbalizes the importance of avoiding which actions? Select all that apply.

☐ **1.** Keeping the legs apart while lying in bed

☐ **2.** Periodically tightening the leg muscles

☐ **3.** Internally rotating the feet

☐ **4.** Bending to pick items up from the floor

☐ **5.** Sleeping in a side-lying position

Answer: 3, 4

Rationale: After hip replacement surgery, the client should avoid internally rotating his feet and bending more than 90 degrees. These activities can compromise the hip joint. The client should lie with his legs abducted. Leg-strengthening exercises, such as periodically tightening the leg muscles, are recommended to maintain muscle strength and reduce the risk of thrombus formation. A side-lying position is acceptable; however, some physicians restrict lying on the operative side.

Nursing process step: Evaluation

Client needs category: Physiological integrity

Client needs subcategory: Reduction of risk potential

Cognitive level: Analysis

---

6. A client who was involved in a motor vehicle accident has a fractured femur. The nurse caring for the client identifies *Acute pain* as one of the nursing diagnoses in his care plan. Which nursing interventions are appropriate? Select all that apply.

☐ **1.** Tell the client which pain management option to use.

☐ **2.** Encourage the client to use as little pain medication as possible to avoid addiction.

☐ **3.** Explain that pain management should leave the client pain-free.

☐ **4.** Avoid alternative and supplementary pain control techniques.

☐ **5.** Assess the client's perception of pain.

☐ **6.** Ask the client about methods he previously used to alleviate pain.

Answer: 5, 6

Rationale: The nurse should begin by assessing the client's perception of pain, including characteristics, and methods he previously found effective in managing pain. These interventions provide a baseline from which the nurse can plan interventions and evaluate their success. The nurse should allow the client to decide which pain-control management techniques to use to help increase his self-esteem. Analgesics should be administered as needed to relieve pain. Addiction shouldn't be a concern at this time. After receiving analgesics, the client should indicate that he feels more comfortable by reporting pain as a score of 3 or less on a scale of 0 to 10 (0 being without pain). Being completely pain-free isn't a realistic expectation. The nurse should teach the client alternative and supplementary pain control techniques, such as imagery, distraction, and heat and cold application. These techniques provide the client with options for dealing with pain.

Nursing process step: Implementation

Client needs category: Physiological integrity

Client needs subcategory: Basic care and comfort

Cognitive level: Application

7. A client fractured the neck of his femur in a fall. The nurse is using an illustration to explain to the family where the fracture occurred. Identify the area that the nurse would point out to the family as the site of the fracture.

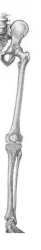

Answer:

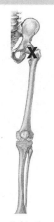

Rationale: The neck of the femur connects the round ball head of the femur to the shaft.

Nursing process step: Implementation

Client needs category: Physiological integrity

Client needs subcategory: Physiological adaptation

Cognitive level: Comprehension

---

8. A nurse is caring for a client with osteomyelitis. The nurse understands the intervention listed on the care plan based on knowledge of which facts about osteomyelitis? Select all that apply.

☐ **1.** Rapidly growing children are most at risk for the disease.

☐ **2.** Liver function enzymes and the erythrocyte sedimentation rate are elevated.

☐ **3.** The disease process is limited to one specific area and doesn't spread.

☐ **4.** Fever and tachycardia are symptoms of the disease.

☐ **5.** Amputation and pathologic fractures may result from the disease process.

☐ **6.** The best treatment includes rapid return to usual activity with the affected area.

Answer: 1, 4, 5

Rationale: Rapidly growing children are most at risk for osteomyelitis but all ages may be affected. Fever and tachycardia along with sudden pain in the affected area accompanied by heat, redness, and swelling are common symptoms of the disease. If the disorder doesn't respond well to treatment or is chronic, pathologic fractures from weakened bone tissue may occur or amputation due to severe pain and functional loss may be necessary. The white blood cell count, not liver enzymes, is elevated as is the sedimentation rate. Osteomyelitis can spread throughout the bone tissues to the periosteum and marrow, and can involve more than one site in the infective process. The best treatment is large doses of I.V. antibiotics, immobilization of the affected area, analgesics, and surgical drainage, if possible.

Nursing process step: Implementation

Client needs category: Physiological integrity

Client needs subcategory: Physiological adaptation

Cognitive level: Application

Neurosensory disorders

1. A client is admitted with a diagnosis of stroke. She has expressive aphasia. Identify the area where the client's stroke has occurred.

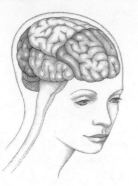

Answer:

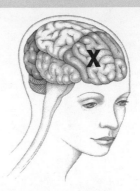

Rationale: The frontal lobe influences language expression as well as personality, judgment, abstract reasoning, social behavior, and movement.

Nursing process step: Data collection

Client needs category: Physiological integrity

Client needs subcategory: Physiologic adaptation

Cognitive level: Comprehension

---

2. A client is experiencing vision disturbances and is diagnosed with cataracts. Identify the area of the eye that's diseased.

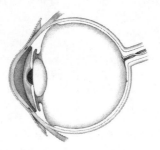

Answer:

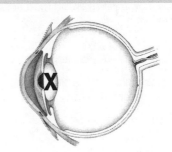

Rationale: The lens is clouded and opaque in cataracts.

Nursing process step: Data collection

Client needs category: Physiological integrity

Client needs subcategory: Physiologic adaptation

Cognitive level: Knowledge

3. A nurse is caring for a client with a T5 complete spinal cord injury. The nurse notes flushed skin, diaphoresis above T5, and a blood pressure of 162/96 mm Hg. The client reports a severe, pounding headache. Which nursing interventions would be appropriate for this client? Select all that apply.

☐ **1.** Elevate the head of the bed 90 degrees.

☐ **2.** Loosen constrictive clothing.

☐ **3.** Use a fan to reduce diaphoresis.

☐ **4.** Check for bladder distention and bowel impaction.

☐ **5.** Administer antihypertensive medication as ordered.

☐ **6.** Place the client in a supine position with legs elevated.

Answer: 1, 2, 4, 5

Rationale: The client is exhibiting signs and symptoms of autonomic dysreflexia. The condition is a potentially life-threatening emergency caused by an uninhibited response from the sympathetic nervous system resulting from a lack of control over the autonomic nervous system. The nurse should immediately elevate the head of the bed to 90 degrees and place the extremities in a dependent position to decrease venous return to the heart and increase venous return from the brain. Because tactile stimuli can trigger autonomic dysreflexia, any constrictive clothing should be loosened. The nurse should also check for a distended bladder and bowel impaction—which may trigger autonomic dysreflexia—and correct any problems. Elevated blood pressure is the most life-threatening complication of autonomic dysreflexia because it can cause stroke, myocardial infarction, or seizure activity. If removing the triggering event doesn't reduce the client's blood pressure, I.V. antihypertensives should be administered. A fan shouldn't be used because drafts of cold may trigger autonomic dysreflexia.

Nursing process step: Implementation

Client needs category: Physiological integrity

Client needs subcategory: Reduction of risk potential

Cognitive level: Application

---

4. A nurse is planning care for a client with multiple sclerosis. Which problems should the nurse expect the client to experience? Select all that apply.

☐ **1.** Vision disturbances

☐ **2.** Coagulation abnormalities

☐ **3.** Balance problems

☐ **4.** Immunity compromise

☐ **5.** Mood disorders

Answer: 1, 3, 5

Rationale: Multiple sclerosis, a neuromuscular disorder, may cause vision disturbances, balance problems, and mood disorders. Multiple sclerosis doesn't cause coagulation abnormalities or immunity problems.

Nursing process step: Planning

Client needs category: Physiological integrity

Client needs subcategory: Reduction of risk potential

Cognitive level: Application

5. A nurse examines a client's level of responsiveness. She finds that the client opens his eyes spontaneously, obeys verbal commands, and is oriented to time, place, and person. What's the client's Glasgow Coma Scale score?

Glasgow Coma Scale

Eye opening response

Opens spontaneously = 4
Opens to verbal command = 3
Opens to pain = 2
No response = 1

Best motor response

Obeys verbal commands = 6
Localizes painful stimuli = 5
Flexion-withdrawal = 4
Flexion-abnormal (decorticate rigidity) = 3
Extension (decerebrate rigidity) = 1

Best verbal response

Oriented and converses = 5
Disoriented and converses = 4
Inappropriate words = 3
Incomprehensible sounds = 2
No response = 1

Answer: 15

Rationale: The score for spontaneous eye opening is 4; obeying verbal commands, 6; and orientation to time, place and person, 5. The total Glasgow Coma Scale score for this client is 15.

Nursing process step: Data collection

Client needs category: Physiological integrity

Client needs subcategory: Physiological adaptation

Cognitive level: Comprehension

---

6. A client with a history of epilepsy is admitted to the medical-surgical unit. While assisting the client from the bathroom, the nurse observes the start of a tonic-clonic seizure. Which nursing interventions are appropriate for this client? Select all that apply.

☐ **1.** Assist the client to the floor.

☐ **2.** Turn the client to his side.

☐ **3.** Place a pillow under the client's head.

☐ **4.** Give the prescribed dose of oral phenytoin (Dilantin).

☐ **5.** Insert an oral suction device to remove secretions in the mouth.

Answer: 1, 2, 3

Rationale: During a seizure, the nurse should assist the client to the floor to reduce the risk of falling and turn the client on his side to help clear the mouth of oral secretions. If available, it's appropriate to place a pillow under the client's head to protect him from injury. It's inappropriate to introduce anything into the mouth during a seizure because of the risk of choking or compromising the airway; therefore, oral medications and suction devices shouldn't be used.

Nursing process step: Implementation

Client needs category: Physiological integrity

Client needs subcategory: Reduction of risk potential

Cognitive level: Application

7. A nurse is preparing to discuss hearing pathways with a client with a new hearing loss. Place the steps in sound wave transmission that allow an individual to hear in ascending chronological order. Use all the options.

1.	Interpretation of sound by the cerebral cortex
2.	Transmission of vibrations through the air and bone
3.	Stimulation of nerve impulses in the inner ear
4.	Transmission of vibrations to the auditory area of the cerebral cortex

| |
| |
| |
| |

Answer:

2.	Transmission of vibrations through the air and bone
3.	Stimulation of nerve impulses in the inner ear
4.	Transmission of vibrations to the auditory area of the cerebral cortex
1.	Interpretation of sound by the cerebral cortex

Rationale: Vibrations transmitted through air and bone stimulate nerve impulses in the inner ear. The cochlear branch of the acoustic nerve transmits these vibrations to the auditory area of the cerebral cortex. The cerebral cortex then interprets the sound.

Nursing process step: Planning

Client needs category: Physiological integrity

Client needs subcategory: Physiologic adaptation

Cognitive level: Comprehension

---

8. A nurse is assigned to care for a client with early stage Alzheimer's disease. Which nursing interventions should be included in the client's care plan? Select all that apply.

☐ **1.** Make frequent changes in the client's routine.

☐ **2.** Engage the client in complex discussions to improve memory.

☐ **3.** Furnish the client's environment with familiar possessions.

☐ **4.** Assist the client with activities of daily living (ADLs) as necessary.

☐ **5.** Assign tasks in simple steps.

Answer: 3, 4, 5

Rationale: A client with Alzheimer's disease experiences progressive deterioration in cognitive functioning. Familiar possessions may help to orient the client. The client should be encouraged to perform ADLs as much as possible but may need assistance with certain activities. Using a step-by-step approach helps the client complete tasks independently. A client with Alzheimer's disease functions best with consistent routines. Complex discussions don't improve the memory of a client with Alzheimer's disease.

Nursing process step: Planning

Client needs category: Psychosocial integrity

Client needs subcategory: None

Cognitive level: Application

9. A client is admitted to the medical-surgical unit after undergoing intracranial surgery to remove a tumor from the left cerebral hemisphere. Which nursing interventions are appropriate for the client's postoperative care? Select all that apply.

☐ **1.** Place a pillow under the client's head so that his neck is flexed.

☐ **2.** Turn the client on his right side.

☐ **3.** Place pillows under the client's legs to promote hip flexion and venous return.

☐ **4.** Maintain the client in the supine position.

☐ **5.** Apply a soft collar to keep the client's neck in a neutral position.

Rationale: The client should be turned on his right side because lying on the left side would cause the brain to shift into the space previously occupied by the tumor. A soft collar keeps the neck in a neutral position, allowing for adequate perfusion and venous drainage of the brain. Placing a pillow under the head flexes the neck and impairs circulation to the brain. Flexion of the hip increases intracranial pressure and, therefore, is contraindicated. Exclusive use of the supine position isn't indicated.

Nursing process step: Implementation

Client needs category: Physiological integrity

Client needs subcategory: Reduction of risk potential

Cognitive level: Application

---

10. A client is a quadriplegic secondary to a spinal cord injury from a motor vehicle accident. Identify the area of the spinal cord where the injury most likely occurred.

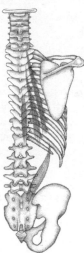

Answer:

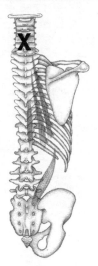

Rationale: Quadriplegia occurs as a result of injury to the cervical segment of the spinal cord.

Nursing process step: Data collection

Client needs category: Physiological integrity

Client needs subcategory: Physiological adaptation

Cognitive level: Comprehension

11. A nurse is reviewing teaching a client with trigeminal neuralgia how to minimize pain episodes. Which comments by the client indicate that he understands the instructions? Select all that apply.

☐ **1.** "I'll eat food that is very hot."

☐ **2.** "I'll try to chew my food on the unaffected side."

☐ **3.** "I can wash my face with cold water."

☐ **4.** "Drinking fluids at room temperature should reduce pain."

☐ **5.** "If tooth brushing is too painful, I'll try to rinse my mouth instead."

Rationale: The facial pain of trigeminal neuralgia is triggered by mechanical or thermal stimuli. Chewing food on the unaffected side and rinsing the mouth rather than brushing teeth reduce mechanical stimulation. Drinking fluids at room temperature reduces thermal stimulation. Eating hot food and washing the face with cold water are likely to trigger pain.

Nursing process step: Evaluation

Client needs category: Health promotion and maintenance

Client needs subcategory: None

Cognitive level: Comprehension

---

12. A client is experiencing problems with balance and fine and gross motor function. Identify that area of the client's brain that's malfunctioning.

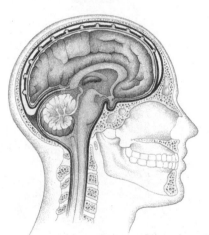

Answer:

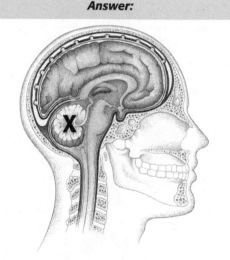

Rationale: The cerebellum is the portion of the brain that controls balance and fine and gross motor function.

Nursing process step: Data collection

Client needs category: Physiological integrity

Client needs subcategory: Reduction of risk potential

Cognitive level: Comprehension

1. A nurse is caring for a client with pneumonia. The physician orders 600 mg of ceftriaxone (Rocephin) oral suspension to be given once per day. The medication label indicates that the strength is 125 mg/5 ml. How many milliliters of medication should the nurse pour to administer the correct dose?

Answer: 24

Rationale: To calculate drug dosages, use the following formula:

Dose on hand/Quantity on hand = Dose desired/X.

In this case:

$$125 \text{ mg/5 ml} = 600 \text{ mg/}X$$

$$X = 24 \text{ ml.}$$

Nursing process step: Implementation

Client needs category: Physiological integrity

Client needs subcategory: Pharmacological therapies

Cognitive level: Application

---

2. A nurse is caring for a client who has a chest tube connected to a three-chamber drainage system without suction. Identify the chamber that collects drainage from the client.

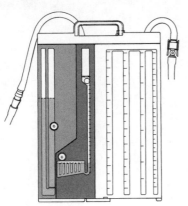

Answer:

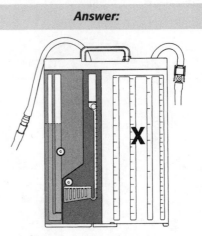

Rationale: The drainage chamber is on the right. It has three calibrated columns showing the amount of drainage collected. When the first column fills, drainage empties into the second; when the second column fills, drainage flows into the third. The water-seal chamber is in the center. The suction-control chamber is on the left.

Nursing process step: Implementation

Client needs category: Physiological integrity

Client needs subcategory: Physiological adaptation

Cognitive level: Comprehension

---

3. A nurse is caring for a client with stage III emphysema. She know that which information about this disorder is correct? Select all that apply.

☐ **1.** Accessory muscle use is often required.

☐ **2.** Continuous high-dose oxygen therapy is required.

☐ **3.** Bronchodilators and corticosteroids are a mainstay of treatment.

☐ **4.** Auscultation reveals normal to decreased breath sounds with wheezes.

☐ **5.** Overdistention and overinflation of the lungs are pathophysiologic findings.

☐ **6.** Influenza vaccination annually and pneumococcal vaccination every 5 years is recommended.

Rationale: Clients with severe emphysema often use accessory muscles to breathe and are more comfortable seated in an upright, slightly tilted forward position. Bronchodilators and corticosteroids are common medications used, with low—not high—dose oxygen therapy to avoid suppressing the respiratory drive. Overdistention and overinflation of the lungs is a key pathophysiologic feature of emphysema. Preventative vaccinations are important to prevent exacerbations by the addition of other lung disease to the preexisting impairment. Auscultation of the chest of the client with emphysema reveals decreased intensity of breath sounds with prolonged expiration.

Nursing process step: Planning

Client needs category: Physiological integrity

Client needs subcategory: Physiological adaptation

Cognitive level: Analysis

---

4. A nurse is reviewing a staff education module about pulmonary circulation. Trace the path of pulmonary circulation.

| **1.** Pulmonary vein |
| **2.** Right ventricle |
| **3.** Pulmonary artery |
| **4.** Arterioles |
| **5.** Alveoli |
| **6.** Left atrium |

Answer:

| **2.** Right ventricle |
| **3.** Pulmonary artery |
| **4.** Arterioles |
| **5.** Alveoli |
| **1.** Pulmonary vein |
| **6.** Left atrium |

Rationale: The pulmonary artery takes deoxygenated blood from the right side of the heart to the lungs via the arterioles and alveoli. The pulmonary vein carries the oxygenated blood back to the left atrium of the heart for circulation throughout the body.

Nursing process step: Implementation

Client needs category: Physiological integrity

Client needs subcategory: Physiologic adaptation

Cognitive level: Comprehension

5. A nurse observes a pregnant visitor choke on a piece of hot dog in the cafeteria. Place the following steps for removal of a foreign airway obstruction in a pregnant or obese client in ascending chronological order. Use all the options.

1.	Grab fist with other hand and perform backwards thrusts.
2.	Place thumb side of one fist on middle of the client's breastbone.
3.	Encircle the client's chest with both hands under her armpits.
4.	Ask the client if she's choking and needs assistance.
5.	Repeat until foreign body is expelled or the client becomes unresponsive

4.	Ask the client if she's choking and needs assistance.
3.	Encircle the client's chest with both hands under her armpits.
2.	Place thumb side of one fist on middle of the client's breastbone.
1.	Grab fist with other hand and perform backwards thrusts.
5.	Repeat until foreign body is expelled or the client becomes unresponsive

Rationale: Correct hand position provides force for thrusts without internal injury. Thrusts provide force to increase intrathoracic pressure and possibly dislodge the foreign body.

Nursing process step: Implementation

Client needs category: Physiologic integrity

Client needs subcategory: Reduction of risk potential

Cognitive level: Application

---

6. A nurse is caring for a client who's scheduled for a bronchoscopy. Which interventions should the nurse expect to perform to prepare the client for this procedure? Select all that apply.

☐ **1.** Explain the procedure.

☐ **2.** Withhold food and fluids for 2 hours before the test.

☐ **3.** Provide a clear liquid diet for 6 to 12 hours before the test.

☐ **4.** Confirm that a signed informed consent form has been obtained.

☐ **5.** Ask the client to remove his dentures.

☐ **6.** Administer atropine and a sedative.

Rationale: All procedures must be explained to the client in order to obtain informed consent and to reduce anxiety. A signed informed consent form is required for all invasive procedures. Dentures need to be removed for a bronchoscopy because they may become dislodged during the procedure. Atropine is administered before a bronchoscopy to decrease secretions. A sedative may be given to relax the client. Food and fluids are restricted for 6 to 12 hours before the test to avoid the risk of aspiration during the procedure.

Nursing process step: Implementation

Client needs category: Physiological integrity

Client needs subcategory: Reduction of risk potential

Cognitive level: Application

7. A client has just undergone a bronchoscopy. Which nursing interventions are appropriate after this procedure? Select all that apply.

☐ **1.** Keep the client flat for at least 2 hours.

☐ **2.** Provide sips of water to moisten the mouth.

☐ **3.** Withhold food and fluids until the gag reflex returns.

☐ **4.** Assess for hemoptysis and frank bleeding.

☐ **5.** Resume food and fluids when the client's voice returns.

☐ **6.** Monitor the client's vital signs.

Answer: 3, 4, 6

Rationale: To prevent aspiration, the client shouldn't receive food or fluids until his gag reflex returns. Although a small amount of blood in the sputum is expected if a biopsy was performed, frank bleeding indicates hemorrhage and should be reported to the physician immediately. Vital signs should be monitored after the procedure because a vasovagal response may cause bradycardia, laryngospasm can affect respirations, and fever may develop within 24 hours of the procedure. To reduce the risk of aspiration, the client should be placed in a semi-Fowler or side-lying position after the procedure until the gag reflex returns. The client doesn't lose his voice after a bronchoscopy, so voice shouldn't be used as a gauge for resuming food and fluid intake.

Nursing process step: Implementation

Client needs category: Physiological integrity

Client needs subcategory: Reduction of risk potential

Cognitive level: Application

---

8. A nurse is caring for a client with pneumonia. The nurse should expect to observe which signs and symptoms when assessing the client? Select all that apply.

☐ **1.** Dry cough

☐ **2.** Fever

☐ **3.** Bradycardia

☐ **4.** Pericardial friction rub

☐ **5.** Use of accessory muscles during respiration

☐ **6.** Crackles or rhonchi

Answer: 2, 5, 6

Rationale: The client with pneumonia may have a fever, use accessory muscles for breathing, and exhibit crackles or rhonchi on auscultation. Other signs and symptoms of pneumonia include fever, malaise, pleuritic pain, pleural friction rub, dyspnea, tachypnea, tachycardia, and a cough that produces rusty green or bloody sputum (in pneumococcal pneumonia) or yellow-green sputum (in bronchopneumonia). A dry cough, bradycardia, and a pericardial friction rub aren't manifestations of pneumonia.

Nursing process step: Data collection

Client needs category: Physiological integrity

Client needs subcategory: Physiological adaptation

Cognitive level: Application

9. A client is admitted with chronic obstructive pulmonary disease (COPD). Which signs and symptoms are characteristic of COPD? Select all that apply.

☐ **1.** Decreased respiratory rate

☐ **2.** Dyspnea on exertion

☐ **3.** Barrel chest

☐ **4.** Shortened expiratory phase

☐ **5.** Clubbed fingers and toes

☐ **6.** Fever

Answer: 2, 3, 5

Rationale: Typical findings in clients with COPD include dyspnea on exertion, a barrel chest, and clubbed fingers and toes. Clients with COPD are usually tachypneic with a prolonged expiratory phase. Fever is not associated with COPD, unless an infection is also present.

Nursing process step: Data collection

Client needs category: Physiological integrity

Client needs subcategory: Physiological adaptation

Cognitive level: Comprehension

---

10. A client is prescribed continuous positive airway pressure (CPAP) therapy for sleep apnea. The nurse instructs the client about the mechanism designed to maintain positive end-expiratory pressure. Identify the area where this mechanism is located.

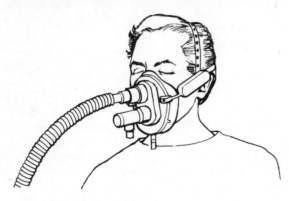

Answer:

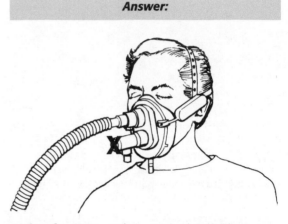

Rationale: CPAP ventilation maintains positive pressure in the airways throughout the client's respiratory cycle. The inlet valve attaches the oxygen tubing to the facemask; the positive end-expiratory pressure valve maintains the pressure and is located as shown. CPAP can be used with or without a ventilator in intubated and nonintubated clients, and can be administered nasally only for a less constrictive feeling by the client. In additon to sleep apnea, CPAP is used to treat respiratory distress syndrome, pulmonary edema, pulmonary emboli, bronchiolitis, pneumonitis, viral pneumonia, and post-operative atelectasis.

Nursing process step: Implementation

Client needs category: Physiological integrity

Client needs subcategory: Physiological adaptation

Cognitive level: Application

---

11. A nurse is about to perform nasopharyngeal suctioning on a client who recently had a stroke. Identify the area where the tip of the suction catheter should be placed.

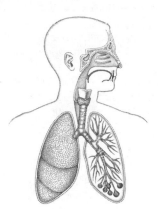

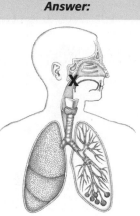

Rationale: When performing nasopharyngeal suctioning, the tip of the catheter is introduced into the naris and advanced to the pharynx. The tip remains above the posterior wall of the mouth.

Nursing process step: Implementation

Client needs category: Physiological integrity

Client needs subcategory: Physiological adaptation

Cognitive level: Application

---

12. The nurse is caring for a client with tuberculosis. Which precautions should the nurse take when providing care for this client? Select all that apply.

☐ **1.** Wear gloves when handling tissues containing sputum.

☐ **2.** Wear a face mask at all times.

☐ **3.** When the client leaves the room for tests, have all people in contact with him wear a mask.

☐ **4.** Keep the client's door open to allow fresh air into the room and prevent social isolation.

☐ **5.** Wash hands after direct contact with the client or contaminated articles.

Answer: 1, 2, 6

Rationale: The nurse should always wear gloves when handling items contaminated with sputum or body secretions. All staff and visitors must wear face masks when coming in contact with the client in his room; masks must be discarded before leaving the client's room. Hand washing is required after direct contact with the client or contaminated articles. The client, not the people in contact with him, must wear a mask when leaving the room for tests. The client should be in a negative-pressure, private room, and the door should remain closed at all times to prevent the spread of infection.

Nursing process step: Implementation

Client needs category: Safe, effective care environment

Client needs subcategory: Safety and infection control

Cognitive level: Application

Genitourinary disorders

1. A nurse is checking a client who has a urinary tract infection (UTI). Which statements should the nurse expect the client to make? Select all that apply.

☐ **1.** "I urinate large amounts."

☐ **2.** "I need to urinate frequently."

☐ **3.** "It burns when I urinate."

☐ **4.** "My urine smells sweet."

☐ **5.** "I need to urinate urgently."

Rationale: Typical findings for a client with a UTI include urinary frequency, burning on urination, and urinary urgency. The client with a UTI typically reports that he voids frequently in small amounts, not large amounts. The client with a UTI complains of foul-smelling, not sweet-smelling, urine.

Nursing process step: Data collection

Client needs category: Physiological integrity

Client needs subcategory: Physiological adaptation

Cognitive level: Application

---

2. A nurse is reviewing the procedure for how to collect a 24-hour urine specimen for creatinine clearance with the client. Which directions should the nurse give the client? Select all that apply.

☐ **1.** "Save the first voiding and record the time."

☐ **2.** "Discard the first voiding and record the time."

☐ **3.** "Clean the perineal area before each voiding."

☐ **4.** "Refrigerate the urine sample or keep it on ice."

☐ **5.** "At the end of 24 hours, void and save the urine."

☐ **6.** "At the end of 24 hours, void and discard the urine."

Answer: 2, 4, 5

Rationale: When collecting a 24-hour urine sample, the client should void, discard the urine, and record the time. This assures that the client starts the collection period with an empty bladder. At the end of the 24-hour collection period, the client should void and save the urine. The first voiding is not used because it isn't known how long the urine has been in the bladder. The urine sample should be refrigerated or kept on ice to keep it fresh. The perineum should be cleaned before obtaining a clean-catch urine specimen for culture and sensitivity. It isn't necessary to clean the perineum for a 24-hour urine sample.

Nursing process step: Implementation

Client needs category: Physiological integrity

Client needs subcategory: Reduction of risk potential

Cognitive level: Application

3. A nurse is caring for a client with chronic renal failure. The laboratory results indicate hypocalcemia and hyperphosphatemia. When checking the client, the nurse should be alert for which signs and symptoms? Select all that apply.

☐ **1.** Trousseau's sign

☐ **2.** Cardiac arrhythmias

☐ **3.** Constipation

☐ **4.** Decreased clotting time

☐ **5.** Drowsiness and lethargy

☐ **6.** Fractures

Rationale: Hypocalcemia is a calcium deficit that causes nerve fiber irritability and repetitive muscle spasms. Signs and symptoms of hypocalcemia include Trousseau's sign, cardiac arrhythmias, diarrhea, increased clotting times, anxiety, and irritability. The calcium-phosphorus imbalance leads to brittle bones and pathologic fractures.

Nursing process step: Data collection

Client needs category: Physiological integrity

Client needs subcategory: Reduction of risk potential

Cognitive level: Application

---

4. A client is diagnosed with renal calculi and complains of severe left flank pain. Scans indicate the calculi are lodged in the left renal pelvis. Identify the structure where the renal calculi are located.

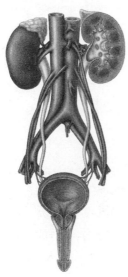

Answer:

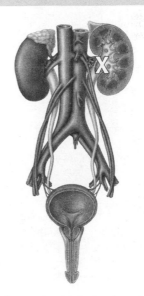

Rationale: The renal pelvis is the area that receives the urine through the major calyces. It receives the urine because it's the widened proximal end of the ureter.

Nursing process step: Data collection

Client needs category: Physiological integrity

Client needs subcategory: Physiologic adaptation

Cognitive level: Application

A nurse is caring for a client with a cystostomy for urine drainage. Identify the area where the nurse should check for cystostomy placement.

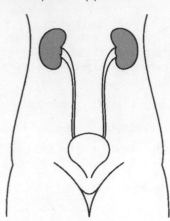

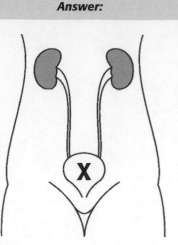

Rationale: In a cystostomy, a catheter is inserted percutaneously through the suprapubic area into the bladder.

Nursing process step: Data collection

Client needs category: Physiological integrity

Client needs subcategory: Basic care and comfort

Cognitive level: Comprehension

---

6. A nurse is completing an intake and output record for a client who is receiving continuous bladder irrigation after transurethral resection of the prostate. How many milliliters of urine should the nurse record as output for her shift if the client received 1,800 ml of normal saline irrigating solution and the output in the urine drainage bag is 2,400 ml?

Answer: 600

Rationale: To calculate urine output, subtract the amount of irrigation solution infused into the bladder from the total amount of fluid in the drainage bag (2,400 ml − 1,800 ml = 600 ml).

Nursing process step: Data collection

Client needs category: Physiological integrity

Client needs subcategory: Reduction of risk potential

Cognitive level: Application

PART THREE

Maternal-infant nursing

1. A client comes to the office for her first prenatal visit. She reports that October 5 was the first day of her last menstrual period. Which statements represent findings in the first trimester of pregnancy? Select all that apply.

☐ **1.** Slow fetal cell differentiation is occurring.

☐ **2.** The client's estimated date of delivery is June 12.

☐ **3.** The client may expect to have some nausea and increased urinary frequency.

☐ **4.** The client will notice decreased vaginal secretions.

☐ **5.** The client's breasts may become swollen and tender.

☐ **6.** Chadwick's sign will be positive at 9 weeks.

Answer: 3, 5, 6

Rationale: The client can expect to have nausea, possible vomiting, urinary frequency, and swollen, tender breasts in the first trimester. Bluish discoloration of the mucous membranes of the vagina, cervix, and vulva (Chadwick's sign) can be noticed beginning at 9 weeks. There's rapid fetal cell differentiation occurring and the client may expect increased—not decreased—vaginal secretions. The estimated date of delivery is calculated using Nägele's rule; thus October 5 - 3 months = July 5; + 7 days makes the date July 12, not June 12.

Nursing process step: Planning

Client needs category: Health promotion and maintenance

Client needs subcategory: None

Cognitive level: Analysis

2. A nurse is assisting with a prenatal assessment on a client who is 32 weeks pregnant. She performs Leopold's maneuvers and determines that the fetus is in the cephalic position. Identify the area where the nurse should place the Doppler to auscultate fetal heart tones.

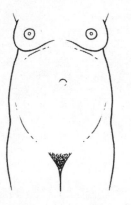

Answer:

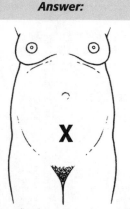

Rationale: When the fetus is in the cephalic position, fetal heart tones are best auscultated midway between the symphysis pubis and the umbilicus. When the fetus is in the breech position, fetal heart tones are best heard at or above the level of the umbilicus.

Nursing process step: Data collection

Client needs category: Health promotion and maintenance

Client needs subcategory: None

Cognitive level: Analysis

3. A client comes to the office for her first prenatal visit. She asks the nurse what physiological changes she can expect during pregnancy. The nurse knows that changes can be in three categories: presumptive, probable, and positive. The nurse prepares to start the discussion with the probable changes of pregnancy. Put the following probable changes in ascending chronological order. Use all the options.

1. The vagina changes color from pink to violet (Chadwick's sign); cervix softens (Goodell's sign).

2. Serum laboratory tests are positive for human chorionic gonadotropin.

3. Braxton Hicks contractions and fetal outline can be palpated through the abdomen.

4. Fetus can be felt to rise against the abdominal wall when lower uterine segment is tapped during a bimanual examination (Ballottement).

Answer:

2. Serum laboratory tests are positive for human chorionic gonadotropin.

1. The vagina changes color from pink to violet (Chadwick's sign); cervix softens (Goodell's sign).

4. Fetus can be felt to rise against the abdominal wall when lower uterine segment is tapped during a bimanual examination (Ballottement).

3. Braxton Hicks contractions and fetal outline can be palpated through the abdomen.

Rationale: Probable changes that strongly suggest pregnancy include laboratory tests, which are positive at about 1 week from implantation. Chadwick's and Goodell's signs occur at 6 weeks. Ballottement occurs at 16 weeks. Braxton Hicks contractions and palpation of the fetal outline can occur as early as 20 weeks.

Nursing process step: Planning

Client needs category: Health promotion and maintenance

Client needs subcategory: None

Cognitive level: Application

---

4. Which nutritional instructions should the nurse review with a 32-year-old primigravida? Select all that apply.

- ☐ **1.** Caloric intake should be increased by 300 cal/day.
- ☐ **2.** Protein intake should be increased to more than 30 g/day.
- ☐ **3.** Vitamin intake should not increase from prepregnancy requirements.
- ☐ **4.** Folic acid intake should be increased to 400 mg/day.
- ☐ **5.** Intake of all minerals, especially iron, should be increased.

Answer: 1, 2, 5

Rationale: A pregnant woman should increase her caloric intake by 300 cal/day. The protein requirements (76 g/day) of a pregnant woman exceed those of a nonpregnant woman by 30 g/day. All mineral requirements, especially iron, are increased in a pregnant woman. The woman should increase her intake of all vitamins and a prenatal vitamin is usually recommended. Folic acid intake is particularly important to help prevent fetal anomalies such as neural tube defect. Intake should be increased from 400 to 800 mg/day.

Nursing process step: Planning

Client needs category: Physiological integrity

Client needs subcategory: Basic care and comfort

Cognitive level: Comprehension

5. During a prenatal screening of a client with diabetes, the nurse should keep in mind that the client is at increased risk for which complications? Select all that apply.

☐ **1.** Still birth

☐ **2.** Rh incompatibility

☐ **3.** Gestational hypertension

☐ **4.** Placenta previa

☐ **5.** Spontaneous abortion

Rationale: Clients with diabetes are at increased risk for intrauterine fetal death after 36 weeks' gestation. Gestational diabetes is also associated with an increased risk of gestational hypertension and spontaneous abortion. The risk of Rh incompatibility and placenta previa isn't increased in the client with diabetes.

Nursing process step: Data collection

Client needs category: Health promotion and maintenance

Client needs subcategory: None

Cognitive level: Comprehension

---

6. A 30-year-old client comes to the office for a routine prenatal visit. After reading the laboratory test results below, the nurse should prepare the client for which study?

Urine dipstick results	
Date	9/8/06
Time	1320
Initials	JB
Color	yellow
Odor	slightly fruity
Appearance	clear
Specific gravity	1.015
pH	6
Protein	none
Glucose	moderate
Kketones	moderate
Bilirubin	none
Blood	none
Nitrates	none

☐ **1.** Triple screen

☐ **2.** Indirect Coombs' test

☐ **3.** 1-hour glucose tolerance test

☐ **4.** Amniocentesis

Rationale: Screening for gestational diabetes using a 1-hour glucose test is recommended for all pregnant women between 24 and 28 weeks. If the client has a history of previously unexplained fetal loss, family history of diabetes, previous large-for-gestational-age neonate, obesity, or glycosuria, the test should be performed toward the end of the first trimester. The triple screen is a blood study routinely offered between the 15th and 20th week and looks for chromosomal abnormalities. The indirect Coombs' test screens maternal blood for red blood cell antibodies. Amniocentesis is a needle aspiration of fluid from the amniotic sac to detect fetal abnormalities and is usually done between 16 and 18 weeks and after 35 weeks to assess lung maturity.

Nursing process step: Planning

Client needs category: Physiological integrity

Client needs subcategory: Reduction of risk potential

Cognitive level: Application

7. Which signs are considered presumptive signs of pregnancy? Select all that apply.

☐ **1.** Goodell's sign

☐ **2.** Uterine enlargement

☐ **3.** Ballottement

☐ **4.** Nausea and vomiting

☐ **5.** Quickening

☐ **6.** Linea nigra

Rationale: Nausea, vomiting, quickening, and linea nigra are presumtive signs of pregnancy. Goodell's sign, uterine enlargement, and ballottement are all probable signs of pregnancy.

Nursing process step: Data collection

Client needs category: Physiological integrity

Client needs subcategory: Physiological adaptation

Cognitive level: Comprehension

---

8. A nurse is assisting in teaching a 16-year-old pregnant client during a home care visit. The client has complained of fatigue and dyspnea on exertion, and has a low serum iron level. Which information should the nurse expect to be included in the teaching care plan of this client? Select all that apply.

☐ **1.** Eat red meat, green vegetables, eggs, iron-fortified breads, whole grains, and milk.

☐ **2.** Take the iron supplement with milk or an antacid to prevent GI upset.

☐ **3.** Stop taking the iron supplement if constipation occurs.

☐ **4.** If gastric irritation occurs, take the iron supplement on an empty stomach.

☐ **5.** Take the iron supplement with foods containing vitamin C such as orange juice, to enhance absorption.

☐ **6.** Explain that pregnancy increases the body's need for iron.

Rationale: The client should be taught a well-balanced diet, such as red meat, green vegetables, eggs, iron-fortified breads, whole grains, and milk, and she should be taught to increase her vitamin C intake because acidity enhances the absorption of iron supplements. The mother and fetus require extra iron, so dietary sources may not be sufficient during pregnancy to prevent iron deficiency anemia. Milk or antacids taken with iron supplements will interfere with absorption by decreasing gastric acidity. Iron supplements should be a continuing therapy because replacement of iron stores takes time. If constipation occurs, high-fiber foods should be increased. If gastric irritation occurs, the client may take iron with food.

Nursing process step: Implementation

Client needs category: Physiological integrity

Client needs subcategory: Pharmacological therapies

Cognitive level: Application

9. A client with hyperemesis gravidarum is on a clear liquid diet. Which foods would be appropriate for the nurse to serve? Select all that apply.

☐ **1.** Milk and ice chips

☐ **2.** Decaffeinated coffee and scrambled eggs

☐ **3.** Tea and gelatin

☐ **4.** Ginger ale and apple juice

☐ **5.** Cranberry juice and chicken broth

☐ **6.** Oatmeal and egg substitutes

Answer: 3, 4, 5

Rationale: A clear liquid diet consists of foods that are clear liquids at room temperature or body temperature, such as ice pops, regular or decaffeinated coffee and tea, gelatin desserts, broth, carbonated beverages, and clear juices, such as apple and cranberry juices. Milk, pasteurized eggs, egg substitutes, and oatmeal are part of a full liquid diet.

Nursing process step: Implementation

Client needs category: Physiological integrity

Client needs subcategory: Basic care and comfort

Cognitive level: Comprehension

---

10. A nurse is palpating the uterus of a client who's 20 weeks pregnant in order to measure fundal height. Identify the area on the abdomen where the nurse should expect to feel the uterine fundus.

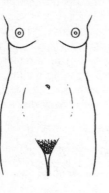

Answer:

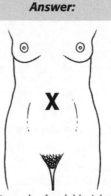

Rationale: At 20 weeks, fundal height should be at approximately the umbilicus. Fundal height should be measured from the symphysis pubis to the top of the uterus (McDonald's Method). Serial measurements assess fetal growth over the course of the pregnancy. Between weeks 18 and 30, the centimeters measured correlate approximately with the week of gestation. However, if the woman is very tall or very short, fundal height will differ.

Nursing process step: Data collection

Client needs category: Health promotion and maintenance

Client needs subcategory: None

Cognitive level: Application

11. A nurse is taking a course on the anatomy and physiology of reproduction. In the illustration of the female reproductive organs, identify the area where fertilization occurs.

Answer:

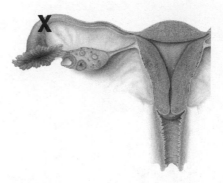

Rationale: After ejaculation, the sperm travel by flagellar movement through the fluids of the cervical mucus into the fallopian tube to meet the descending ovum in the ampulla. This is where fertilization occurs.

Nursing process step: Implementation

Client needs category: Health promotion and maintenance

Client needs subcategory: None

Cognitive level: Application

---

12. A client is scheduled for amniocentesis. What should the nurse do to prepare the client for the procedure? Select all that apply.

☐ **1.** Ask the client to void.

☐ **2.** Instruct the client to drink 1 L of fluid.

☐ **3.** Ask the client to lie on her left side.

☐ **4.** Determine fetal heart rate.

☐ **5.** Insert an I.V. catheter.

☐ **6.** Monitor maternal vital signs.

Answer: 1, 4, 6

Rationale: To prepare a client for amniocentesis, the nurse should ask the client to empty her bladder to reduce the risk of bladder perforation. Before the procedure, the nurse should also determine fetal heart rate and maternal vital signs to establish baselines. The client should be asked to drink 1 L of fluid before transabdominal ultrasound, not amniocentesis. The client should be supine during the procedure; afterward, she should be placed on her left side to avoid supine hypotension, to promote venous return, and to ensure adequate cardiac output. I.V. access isn't necessary for this procedure.

Nursing process step: Implementation

Client needs category: Physiological integrity

Client needs subcategory: Reduction of risk potential

Cognitive level: Application

13. In early pregnancy, some clients complain of abdominal pain or pulling. Identify the area most commonly associated with this pain.

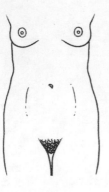

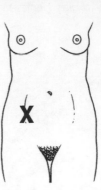

Rationale: As the uterus grows in early pregnancy, it deviates physically to the right. This shift, or dextrorotation, is due to the presence of the rectosigmoid colon in the left lower quadrant. As a result, many women complain of pain in the right lower quadrant.

Nursing process step: Data collection

Client needs category: Health promotion and maintenance

Client needs subcategory: None

Cognitive level: Analysis

Intrapartum period

1. A nurse is assisting in monitoring a client who's receiving oxytocin (Pitocin) to induce labor. The nurse should be alert to which maternal adverse reactions? Select all that apply.

☐ **1.** Hypertension

☐ **2.** Jaundice

☐ **3.** Dehydration

☐ **4.** Fluid overload

☐ **5.** Uterine tetany

☐ **6.** Bradycardia

Answer: 1, 4, 5

Rationale: Adverse effects of oxytocin in the mother include hypertension, fluid overload, and uterine tetany. Oxytocin's antidiuretic effect increases renal reabsorption of water, leading to fluid overload — not dehydration. Jaundice and bradycardia are adverse effects that may occur in the neonate. Tachycardia — not bradycardia — is reported as a maternal adverse effect.

Nursing process step: Data collection

Client needs category: Physiological integrity

Client needs subcategory: Pharmacological therapies

Cognitive level: Application

2. A client is being admitted to the labor and delivery unit. She's GTPAL 5-2-1-1-2. Which statements are true about this client? Select all that apply.

- ☐ **1.** The client has had 4 previous pregnancies.

- ☐ **2.** The client has had 5 previous pregnancies.

- ☐ **3.** The client has had 1 full-term child, 1 abortion, and 1 premature child.

- ☐ **4.** The client has had 2 full-term children, 1 premature child, and 1 abortion.

- ☐ **5.** The client has 3 living children and is pregnant again.

- ☐ **6.** The client has 2 living children and is pregnant again.

Answer: 1, 4, 6

Rationale: Detailed information about a client's obstetric history is described using the GTPAL classification system. G represents *gravida* or the number of times the client has been pregnant, including the current pregnancy. T is the number of full-term infants born (after 37 weeks), P is the number of preterm infants born (before 37 weeks), A is the number of induced or spontaneous abortions, and L is the number of living children.

Nursing process step: Data collection

Client needs category: Health promotion and maintenance

Client needs subcategory: None

Cognitive Level: Application

---

3. A nurse is assisting in the evaluation of a client who's 34 weeks pregnant for premature rupture of the membranes (PROM). Which findings indicate that PROM has occurred? Select all that apply.

- ☐ **1.** Fernlike pattern when vaginal fluid is placed on a glass slide and allowed to dry

- ☐ **2.** Acidic pH of fluid when tested with nitrazine paper

- ☐ **3.** Presence of amniotic fluid in the vagina

- ☐ **4.** Cervical dilation of 6 cm

- ☐ **5.** Alkaline pH of fluid when tested with nitrazine paper

- ☐ **6.** Contractions occurring every 5 minutes

Answer: 1, 3, 5

Rationale: The fernlike pattern that occurs when vaginal fluid is placed on a glass slide and allowed to dry, presence of amniotic fluid in the vagina, and alkaline pH of fluid are all signs of ruptured membranes. The fernlike pattern is a result of the high sodium and protein content of the amniotic fluid. The presence of amniotic fluid in the vagina results from the expulsion of the fluid from the amniotic sac. Cervical dilation and regular contractions are signs of progressing labor but do not indicate PROM.

Nursing process step: Data collection

Client needs category: Physiological integrity

Client needs subcategory: Physiological adaptation

Cognitive level: Analysis

4. A nurse is caring for a client who has been diagnosed with abruptio placentae. What signs and symptoms of abruptio placentae should the nurse expect to find when she's collecting data on this client? Select all that apply.

☐ **1.** Vaginal bleeding

☐ **2.** Decreased fundal height

☐ **3.** Uterine tenderness on palpation

☐ **4.** Soft abdomen on palpation

☐ **5.** Hypotonic, small uterus

☐ **6.** Abnormal fetal heart tones

Answer: 1, 3, 6

Rationale: Painful vaginal bleeding, uterine tenderness on palpation, and abnormal or absent heart tones are signs of abruptio placentae. Fundal height increases during abruptio placentae as a result of blood becoming trapped behind the placenta. The abdomen would feel hard and boardlike on palpation as blood permeates the myometrium and causes uterine irritability. The uterus would also be hypertonic and enlarged.

Nursing process step: Data collection

Client needs category: Physiological integrity

Client needs subcategory: Physiological adaptation

Cognitive level: Comprehension

---

5. A client who's 29 weeks pregnant comes to the labor and delivery unit. She states that she's having contractions every 8 minutes. The client is also 3 cm dilated. Which treatments can the nurse expect to administer? Select all that apply.

☐ **1.** Folic acid (Folvite)

☐ **2.** Terbutaline (Brethine)

☐ **3.** Betamethasone

☐ **4.** Rh_o (D) immune globulin (Rhogam)

☐ **5.** I.V. fluids

☐ **6.** Meperidine (Demerol)

Answer: 2, 3, 5

Rationale: The client is at risk for preterm delivery. The nurse can expect that terbutaline, a beta$_2$-adrenergic agonist that relaxes smooth muscle, will be administered to halt contractions. The nurse can also expect that betamethasone, a corticosteroid, will be administered to decrease the risk of respiratory distress in the infant if preterm delivery occurs. I.V. fluids will be used to expand the intravascular volume and decrease contractions, if dehydration is the cause. Folic acid is a mineral recommended throughout pregnancy (especially in the first trimester) to decrease the risk of neural tube defects. It isn't used to address preterm delivery. Rh_o (D) immune globulin is administered to Rh-negative clients who have been or are suspected of having been exposed to Rh-positive fetal blood. Meperidine is an opioid used during labor and delivery to manage pain.

Nursing process step: Planning

Client needs category: Physiological integrity

Client needs subcategory: Pharmacological therapies

Cognitive level: Analysis

6. A nurse is assigned to assist with the admission of a client who's in labor. Which actions are appropriate? Select all that apply.

☐ **1.** Asking about the estimated date of delivery (EDD)

☐ **2.** Estimating fetal size

☐ **3.** Taking maternal and fetal vital signs

☐ **4.** Asking about the woman's last menses

☐ **5.** Administering an analgesic

☐ **6.** Asking about the amount of time between contractions

Answer: 1, 3, 6

Rationale: The nurse should ask about the EDD and then compare the response to the information in the prenatal record. If the fetus is preterm, special precautions and equipment are necessary. Maternal and fetal vital signs should be obtained to evaluate the well-being of the client and fetus. Determining how far apart the contractions are provides the health care team with valuable baseline information. The physician estimates the size of the fetus. It wouldn't be appropriate for the nurse to ask about the client's last menses. This information should be collected at the first prenatal visit. It would be premature to administer an analgesic, which could slow or stop labor contractions.

Nursing process step: Implementation

Client needs category: Health promotion and maintenance

Client needs subcategory: None

Cognitive level: Application

---

7. A nurse is assisting in the delivery room. The physician prepares to perform an episiotomy. To do this procedure the physician makes an incision in which part of the client's external genitalia area?

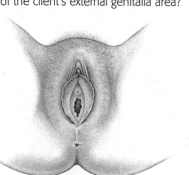

Answer:

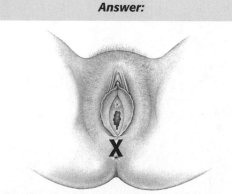

Rationale: An episiotomy is surgical enlargement of the vaginal opening that allows easier delivery of the fetus. The incision is made in the perineum and can be midline or right or left mediolateral.

Nursing process step: Implementation

Client needs category: Physiological integrity

Client needs subcategory: Reduction of risk potential

Cognitive level: Application

8. A nurse is assisting in caring for a client who has just given birth to a neonate through vaginal delivery. The nurse is monitoring for signs of placental separation. Which signs indicate that the placenta has separated? Select all that apply.

☐ **1.** Shortening of the umbilical cord

☐ **2.** Sudden, sharp abdominal pain

☐ **3.** Sudden gush of vaginal blood

☐ **4.** Change in shape of the uterus

☐ **5.** Lengthening of the umbilical cord

Answer: 3, 4, 5

Rationale: Signs of placental separation include lengthening of the umbilical cord, a sudden gush of blood from the vagina, a firmly contracted uterus, and change in uterine shape from discoid to globular. Sudden, sharp abdominal pain could indicate uterine rupture.

Nursing process step: Data collection

Client needs category: Physiological integrity

Client needs subcategory: Physiological adaptation

Cognitive level: Comprehension

---

9. A client in labor is 8 cm dilated and 75% effaced. The fetus, which is in vertex presentation, is at 0 station. In the illustration below, identify the level of the fetus's head.

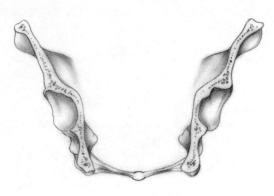

Answer:

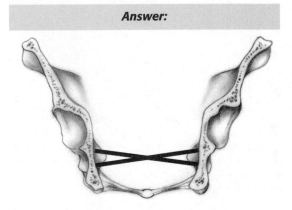

Rationale: Station refers to the level of the presenting part in relation to the pelvic inlet and the ischial spines. A 0 station indicates that the presenting part lies at the level of the ischial spines. Other stations are defined by their distance in centimeters above or below the ischial spines.

Nursing process step: Data collection

Client needs category: Health promotion and maintenance

Client needs subcategory: None

Cognitive level: Application

10. While waiting to receive report at shift change, a nurse reads the chart entry below just written by the previous nurse. After reading this note, the nurse knows her client is in which stage of labor?

> 7/3/06 0135 Client experienced spontaneous rupture of membranes. Fluid is odorless and clear. Contractions are 50 seconds long and occur every 4 minutes. See flow sheet for details. Client is 4 cm dilated. ——
> ——————————————————————A. Wilkens, LPN

☐ **1.** Stage 1, latent phase

☐ **2.** Stage 2

☐ **3.** Stage 1, active phase

☐ **4.** Stage 1, transition phase

Answer: 3

Rationale: During the active phase of stage 1 of labor, membranes may rupture spontaneously. Contractions last about 40 to 60 seconds and recur every 3 to 5 minutes, and the cervix dilates from about 3 to 7 cm. During the latent phase of stage 1, contractions last 20 to 40 seconds and occur every 5 to 30 minutes, and the cervix dilates from 0 to 3 cm. During stage 2 of labor, the cervix is fully dilated and effaced and the neonate is born. During the transition phase of stage 1, contractions last 60 to 90 seconds and occur every 2 to 3 minutes, and the cervix dilates from 7 cm to fully dilated at 10 cm.

Nursing process step: Evaluation

Client needs category: Safe and effective care environment

Client needs subcategory: Coordinated care

Cognitive level: Application

Postpartum period

1. On examining a client who gave birth 3 hours ago, a nurse finds that the client has completely saturated a perineal pad within 15 minutes. Which actions should the nurse take? Select all that apply.

☐ **1.** Begin an I.V. infusion of lactated Ringer's solution.

☐ **2.** Assess the client's vital signs.

☐ **3.** Palpate the client's fundus.

☐ **4.** Place the client in high Fowler's position.

☐ **5.** Administer a pain medication.

Answer: 2, 3

Rationale: Checking vital signs provides information about the client's circulatory status and identifies significant changes that may need to be reported to the physician. By palpating the client's fundus, the nurse also gains valuable data. A boggy uterus may lead to excessive bleeding. Starting an I.V. infusion requires a physician's order. Placing the client in high Fowler's position may lower the blood pressure and be harmful to the client. Administration of a pain medication does not address the current problem.

Nursing process step: Data collection

Client needs category: Physiological integrity

Client needs subcategory: Reduction of risk potential

Cognitive level: Application

2. A nurse observes several interactions between a mother and her new son. Which behaviors by the mother would the nurse identify as evidence of mother-infant attachment? Select all that apply.

☐ **1.** Talks and coos to her son

☐ **2.** Cuddles her son close to her

☐ **3.** Doesn't make eye contact with her son

☐ **4.** Requests the nurse to take the baby to the nursery for feedings

☐ **5.** Encourages the father to hold the baby

☐ **6.** Takes a nap when the baby is sleeping

Answer: 1, 2

Rationale: Talking to, cooing to, and cuddling with her son are positive signs that the mother is adapting to her new role. Avoiding eye contact is a sign that the mother is not bonding with her baby. Eye contact, touching, and speaking are important to establish attachment with an infant. Feeding a neonate is an important role of a new mother and facilitates attachment. Encouraging the dad to hold the baby facilitates attachment between the neonate and the father. Resting while the infant is sleeping conserves needed energy and allows the mother to be alert and awake when her infant is awake; however, it isn't evidence of bonding.

Nursing process step: Evaluation

Client needs category: Psychosocial integrity

Client needs subcategory: None

Cognitive level: Analysis

---

3. A mother with a history of varicose veins has just delivered her first baby. The nurse suspects that the mother has developed a pulmonary embolus. Which data would lead to this nursing judgment? Select all that apply.

☐ **1.** Sudden dyspnea

☐ **2.** Chills, fever

☐ **3.** Diaphoresis

☐ **4.** Hypertension

☐ **5.** Confusion

Answer: 1, 3, 5

Rationale: Sudden dyspnea with diaphoresis and confusion are classic signs and symptoms of dislodgment of a thrombus (stationary blood clot) from a varicose vein. The thrombus becomes an embolus (moving clot) that lodges itself in the pulmonary circulation. Chills and fever would indicate an infection. A client with an embolus could be hypotensive, not hypertensive.

Nursing process step: Data collection

Client needs category: Physiological integrity

Client needs subcategory: Physiological adaptation

Cognitive level: Analysis

4. On a client's second postpartum visit, the physician reviews the chart below regarding the client's lochia. What's the best term for the lochia described?

Lochia		
Date	10-12-06	10-13-06
Time	0945	0930
Color	Red	Red
Odor	Normal	Normal
Consistency	Few tiny clots	No clots
Amount	4 pads/24 hr	3 pads/24 hr

☐ **1.** Alba

☐ **2.** Thrombic

☐ **3.** Serosa

☐ **4.** Rubra

Answer: 4

Rationale: Lochia rubra is a red discharge that occurs 1 to 3 days after birth. It consists almost entirely of blood with only small clots and mucus. Lochia alba is a creamy white or colorless discharge that occurs 10 to 14 days postpartum and may continue for up to 6 weeks. Lochia serosa is a pink or brownish discharge that occurs 4 to 10 days postpartum. Lochia thrombic isn't a valid term.

Nursing process step: Data collection

Client needs category: Physiological integrity

Client needs subcategory: Physiological adaptation

Cognitive level: Application

---

5. A nurse is caring for a 1-day postpartum mother. Reading the progress note below (from the previous shift), the nurse notes that the mother is in which phase of the postpartum period?

> Mother verbalizing labor and delivery experience. Does not appear confident in holding baby or with diaper changes. Asking questions appropriately.
> ————————————————————J. Conners, LP

☐ **1.** Letting-go

☐ **2.** Taking-in

☐ **3.** Holding-out

☐ **4.** Taking-hold

Answer: 2

Rationale: The taking-in phase is a normal first phase for a mother when she's feeling overwhelmed by the responsibilities of neonatal care while still fatigued from delivery. Taking hold is the next phase, when the mother has rested and she can think and learn mothering skills with confidence. Letting go is the final stage, when the mother adapts to parenthood, her new definition as a caregiver, and her new baby as a separate entity. Holding out isn't a valid stage.

Nursing process step: Data collection

Client needs category: Psychosocial integrity

Client needs subcategory: None

Cognitive level: Analysis

6. A client has received treatment for a warm, reddened, painful area in the breast as well as cracked and fissured nipples. The client expresses the desire to continue breast-feeding. Which interventions should the nurse expect to see on the care plan to prevent a recurrence of the problem? Select all that apply.

☐ **1.** Wash the nipples with soap and water.

☐ **2.** Change the breast pads frequently.

☐ **3.** Expose the nipples to air for part of each day.

☐ **4.** Wash hands before handling the breast and breast-feeding.

☐ **5.** Make sure that the baby grasps the nipple only.

☐ **6.** Release the baby's grasp on the nipple before removing the baby from the breast.

Answer: 2, 3, 4, 6

Rationale: Because mastitis is an infection frequently associated with a break in the skin surface of the nipple, measures to prevent cracked and fissured nipples help prevent it. Changing breast pads frequently and exposing the nipples to air for part of the day help keep the nipples dry and prevent irritation. Washing hands before handling the breast reduces the chance of accidentally introducing organisms into the breast. Releasing the baby's grasp on the nipple before removing the baby from the breast also reduces the chance of irritation. Nipples should be washed with water only; soap tends to remove the natural oils and increases the chance of cracking. The baby should grasp both the nipple and areola.

Nursing process step: Planning

Client needs category: Physiological integrity

Client needs subcategory: Physiological adaptation

Cognitive level: Analysis

---

7. A nurse is caring for a postpartum client suspected of developing postpartum psychosis. Which statements accurately characterize this disorder? Select all that apply.

☐ **1.** Symptoms start 2 days after delivery.

☐ **2.** The disorder is common in postpartum women.

☐ **3.** Symptoms include delusions and hallucinations.

☐ **4.** Suicide and infanticide are uncommon in this disorder.

☐ **5.** The disorder rarely occurs without psychiatric history.

Answer: 3, 5

Rationale: Psychosis should be suspected in a postpartum woman if she exhibits manic-depressive behaviors (delusions or hallucinations with symptoms, such as restlessness and insomnia, irritability, rapidly shifting moods, and disorganized behavior), generally starting within 2 weeks of delivery. Typically, the woman has a history of a psychiatric disorder or previous postpartum psychosis. A history of bipolar disorder is an important risk factor. The disorder occurs in less than 1% of postpartum mothers and it's considered a medical emergency. Suicide is common and infanticide occurs in up to 4% of clients with the disorder.

Nursing process step: Data collection

Client needs category: Physiological integrity

Client needs subcategory: Reduction of risk potential

Cognitive level: Analysis

8. A nurse is palpating the uterine fundus of a client who delivered 8 hours ago. Identify the area of the abdomen where the nurse would expect to feel the fundus.

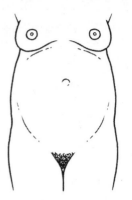

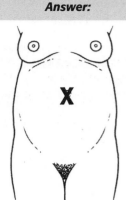

Rationale: The nurse should be able to feel the uterus at the level of the umbilicus from 1 hour after birth to approximately 24 hours after birth.

Nursing process step: Data collection

Client needs category: Physiological integrity

Client needs subcategory: Reduction of risk potential

Cognitive level: Comprehension

---

9. A nurse is assisting in developing a care plan for a client with an episiotomy. Which interventions would be included for the nursing diagnosis *Acute pain related to perineal sutures*? Select all that apply.

☐ **1.** Apply an ice pack intermittently to the perineal area for 3 days.

☐ **2.** Avoid the use of topical pain gels.

☐ **3.** Administer sitz baths three to four times per day.

☐ **4.** Encourage the client to do Kegel exercises.

☐ **5.** Limit the number of times the perineal pad is changed.

Answer: 3, 4

Rationale: Sitz baths help decrease inflammation and tension in the perineal area. Kegel exercises improve circulation to the area and help reduce edema. Ice packs should be applied to the perineum for only the first 24 hours; after that time, heat should be used. Topical pain gels should be applied to the suture area to reduce discomfort, as ordered. The perineal pad should be changed frequently to prevent irritation caused by the discharge.

Nursing process step: Planning

Client needs category: Physiological integrity

Client needs subcategory: Basic care and comfort

Cognitive level: Application

The neonate

1. A nurse is administering vitamin K to a neonate after delivery. The medication is supplied in a concentration of 2 mg/ml and the ordered dose is 0.5 mg subcutaneously. How many milliliters should the nurse administer?

_____

Answer: 0.25

Rationale: Use the following formula to calculate this dose:

$$\text{Dose on hand/Quantity on hand} = \text{Desired dose}/X$$

$$2 \text{ mg/ml} = 0.5 \text{ mg}/X$$

$$X = 0.25 \text{ ml.}$$

Nursing process step: Implementation

Client needs category: Physiological integrity

Client needs subcategory: Pharmacological therapies

Cognitive level: Analysis

---

2. A 14-day-old neonate is admitted for aspiration pneumonia. The results of a barium swallow confirm a diagnosis of gastroesophageal reflux with resulting aspiration pneumonia. Identify the area of the stomach that's weakened, contributing to the reflux.

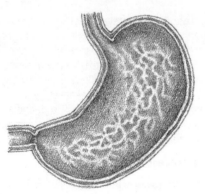

Answer:

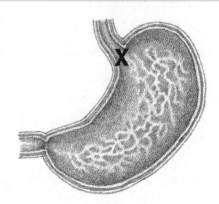

Rationale: Gastroesophageal reflux is a neuromotor disturbance in which the cardiac sphincter is lax and allows easy regurgitation of gastric contents into the esophagus, causing possible aspiration into the lungs. The cardiac sphincter is located between the stomach and the esophagus.

Nursing process step: Data collection

Client needs category: Physiological integrity

Client needs subcategory: Physiological adaptation

Cognitive level: Comprehension

3. In the nursery, a nurse is performing a neurologic examination on a 1-day-old neonate. Which findings would indicate possible asphyxia in utero? Select all that apply.

☐ **1.** The neonate grasps the nurse's finger when she puts it in the palm of his hand.

☐ **2.** The neonate does stepping movements when held upright with his sole touching a surface.

☐ **3.** The neonate's toes don't curl downward when his soles are stroked.

☐ **4.** The neonate doesn't respond when the nurse claps her hands above him.

☐ **5.** The neonate turns toward an object when the nurse touches his cheek with it.

☐ **6.** The neonate displays weak, ineffective sucking.

Answer: 3, 4, 6

Rationale: Failure of the toes to curl downward when the soles are stroked and lack of response to a loud sound can be evidence that neurological damage from asphyxia has occurred. The normal responses would be that the toes curl downward with stroking and the arms and legs extend in response to a loud noise. Weak, ineffective sucking is another sign of neurologic damage; a neonate should root and suck when the side of his cheek is stroked. A neonate should also grasp a person's finger when it's placed in the palm of his hand, do stepping movements when held upright with the soles touching a surface, and turn toward an object when his cheek is touched with it.

Nursing process step: Data collection

Client needs category: Health promotion and maintenance

Client needs subcategory: None

Cognitive level: Application

---

4. Which instructions should the nurse expect will be provided on discharge from the facility to the parents of a neonate who has been circumcised? Select all that apply.

☐ **1.** The infant must void before being discharged home.

☐ **2.** Apply petroleum jelly to the glans of the penis with each diaper change.

☐ **3.** Tub baths for the infant are acceptable while the circumcision heals.

☐ **4.** Report any blood on the front of the diaper.

☐ **5.** The circumcision requires care for 2 to 4 days after discharge.

Answer: 1, 2, 5

Rationale: It's necessary for a circumcised infant to void before discharge to ensure that the urethra isn't obstructed. A lubricating ointment, such as petroleum jelly, should be applied to the glans with each diaper change. Typically, the penis heals within 2 to 4 days and circumcision care is needed only during that period. Parents should avoid giving the neonate tub baths until the circumcision heals to prevent infection; only sponge baths are appropriate. A small amount of bleeding is expected after circumcision; parents should report only large amounts of bleeding to the physician.

Nursing process step: Implementation

Client needs category: Safe, effective care environment

Client needs subcategory: Coordinated care

Cognitive level: Application

5. A nurse is eliciting reflexes in a neonate during a physical examination. Identify the area the nurse would touch to elicit a plantar grasp reflex.

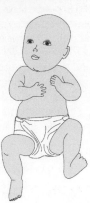

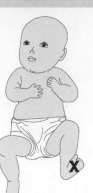

Rationale: Touching the sole of the foot near the base of the digits elicits a plantar grasp reflex and causes flexion or grasping. This reflex disappears around age 9 months.

Nursing process step: Data collection

Client needs category: Health promotion and maintenance

Client needs subcategory: None

Cognitive level: Application

---

6. A nurse is demonstrating cord care to a mother of a neonate. Which actions should the nurse review with the mother? Select all that apply.

☐ **1.** Explain that the diaper is kept below the cord.

☐ **2.** Tug gently on the cord to remove it as it begins to dry.

☐ **3.** Apply antibiotic ointment to the cord twice daily.

☐ **4.** Only sponge-bathe the infant until the cord falls off.

☐ **5.** Clean the length of the cord with alcohol several times daily.

☐ **6.** Wash the cord with mild soap and water.

Answer: 1, 4, 5

Rationale: The diaper should be positioned below the cord to allow for it to air dry and to prevent urine from getting on it. Parents should be instructed to sponge-bathe the infant until the cord falls off; soap and water should not be used. The entire cord should be cleaned with alcohol, using a cotton-tipped applicator or another appropriate method. Parents should also be instructed to never pull on the cord; they should allow it to fall off naturally. Antibiotic ointments are contraindicated unless signs of infection are present.

Nursing process step: Implementation

Client needs category: Safe, effective care environment

Client needs subcategory: Safety and infection control

Cognitive level: Application

7. A nurse notes that at 5 minutes after birth, a neonate is pink with acrocyanosis, has his knees flexed and fists clenched, has a whimpering cry, has a heart rate of 128 beats/minute, and withdraws his foot to a slap on the sole. What 5-minute Apgar score should the nurse record for this neonate?

Sign	Apgar Score		
	0	1	2
Heart rate	Absent	Less than 100 beats/ minute	More than 100 beats/minute
Respirator effort	Absent	Slow, irregular breathing; weak cry	Strong crying, normal rate and breathing
Muscle tone	Flaccid	Some flexion and resistance to extension of extremities	Active motion
Reflex irritability	No response	Grimace	Crying and withdrawal of foot
Color	Pallor, cyanosis	Pink body, blue extremities	Completely normal

Rationale: The Apgar score quantifies neonatal heart rate, respiratory effort, muscle tone, reflexes, irritability, and color. Each category is assessed 1 minute after birth and again 5 minutes later. Scores in each category range from 0 to 2, as shown. This neonate has a heart rate above 100 beats/minute, which equals 2; is pink in color with acrocyanosis, which equals 1; is well-flexed, which equals 2; has a weak cry, which equals 1; and has a good response to slapping the soles, which equals 2. Therefore, the nurse should record a total Apgar score of 8.

Nursing process step: Data collection

Client needs category: Physiological integrity

Client needs subcategory: Physiological adaptation

Cognitive level: Analysis

8. A nurse is providing care to a neonate. List the steps in ascending chronological order to show how opthalmia neonatorum prophylaxis would be performed. Use all the options.

1.	Close and manipulate the eyelids to spread the medication over the eye.
2.	Shield the neonate's eyes from direct light and tilt his head slightly to the side that will receive the treatment.
3.	Repeat the procedure for the other eye.
4.	Wash your hands and put on gloves.
5.	Apply the ointment into the lower conjunctival sac.
6.	Gently raise the neonate's upper eyelid with your index finger and pull the lower eyelid down with your thumb.

Answer:

4.	Wash your hands and put on gloves.
2.	Shield the neonate's eyes from direct light and tilt his head slightly to the side that will receive the treatment.
6.	Gently raise the neonate's upper eyelid with your index finger and pull the lower eyelid down with your thumb.
5.	Apply the ointment into the lower conjunctival sac.
1.	Close and manipulate the eyelids to spread the medication over the eye.
3.	Repeat the procedure for the other eye.

Rationale: Opthalmia neonatorum prophylaxis is the instillation of 0.5% erythromycin ointment or 1% tetracycline ointment into the neonate's eyes to prevent gonorrheal or chlamydial conjunctivitis. Silver nitrate is no longer manufactured in the United States, so it's rarely used today. However, it's the best prophylaxis against known gonorrheal risk. All 50 states mandate that this treatment be given within 1 hour of birth to decrease the risk of permanent eye damage and blindness.

Nursing process step: Implementation

Client needs category: Physiological integrity

Client needs subcategory: Physiological adaptation

Cognitive level: Application

PART FOUR

Pediatric nursing

The infant

1. A physician orders digoxin 0.1 mg orally every morning for a 6-month-old infant with heart failure. Digoxin is available in a 400 mcg/ml concentration. How many milliliters of digoxin should the nurse give?

_____

Answer: 0.25

Rationale: Use the following equations.

To convert mg to mcg:

$$1,000 \text{ mcg}/1 \text{ mg} = X \text{ mcg}/0.1 \text{ mg}$$

$$X = 100 \text{ mcg}.$$

To calculate drug dose:

$$\text{Dose on hand}/\text{Quantity on hand} = \text{Dose desired}/X$$

$$400 \text{ mcg}/\text{ml} = 100 \text{ mcg}/X$$

$$X = 0.25 \text{ ml}.$$

Nursing process step: Implementation

Client needs category: Physiological integrity

Client needs subcategory: Pharmacological therapies

Cognitive level: Application

2. A nurse is checking an infant on a routine visit. The infant coos and babbles after feeding in response to the mother and nurse talking to him, but doesn't smack his lips or make "raspberries." How old is the infant?

☐ **1.** 0 to 2 months

☐ **2.** 3 to 4 months

☐ **3.** 5 to 6 months

☐ **4.** 7 to 9 months

☐ **5.** 10 to 12 months

Answer: 2

Rationale: An infant who coos and babbles in response to someone talking to him is 3 to 4 months old. An infant this age also can respond to the caregiver with a smile. A 0- to 2-month-old infant listens to human voices and produces only vowel sounds. A 5- to 6-month-old infant can make "raspberries" and smack his lips as well as recognize familiar names and sounds. A 7- to 9-month-old infant responds to his name, imitates sounds, and enjoys listening to simple books. A 10- to 12-month-old infant may speak a few words such as "bye-bye" or "ma-ma."

Nursing process step: Data collection

Client needs category: Health promotion and maintenance

Client needs subcategory: None

Cognitive level: Application

3. A nurse has received report on her clients and notices that they are of varying ages. In order to prepare for the shift, the nurse reviews Erikson's five stages of psychosocial development. Place the stages listed below in ascending chronological order starting with infancy, according to Erikson's definitions of infancy, toddlerhood, preschool age, school age, and adolescence. Use all the options.

| **1.** Initiative versus guilt |
| **2.** Trust versus mistrust |
| **3.** Industry versus inferiority |
| **4.** Identity versus role confusion |
| **5.** Autonomy versus shame and doubt |

| |
| |
| |
| |
| |

| **Answer:** |

| **2.** Trust versus mistrust |
| **5.** Autonomy versus shame and doubt |
| **1.** Initiative versus guilt |
| **3.** Industry versus inferiority |
| **4.** Identity versus role confusion |

Rationale: During the first stage of Erikson's five stages of psychosocial development—trust versus mistrust (birth to age 1)—the child develops trust as the primary caregiver meets his needs. In the second stage—autonomy versus shame and doubt (ages 1 to 3)—the child gains control of body functions and becomes increasingly independent. In stage 3—initiative versus guilt (ages 3 to 6)—the child develops a conscience and learns about the world through play. In stage 4—industry versus inferiority (ages 6 to 12)—the child enjoys working on projects with others, follows rules, and forms social relationships. As body changes begin to take place, the child enters stage 5—identity versus role confusion (ages 12 to 19)—and becomes preoccupied with how he looks, how others view him, meeting peer expectations, and establishing his own identity.

Nursing process step: Planning

Client needs category: Health promotion and maintenance

Client needs subcategory: None

Cognitive level: Comprehension

4. A nurse is caring for a 1-month-old infant who fell from the changing table during a diaper change. Which signs and symptoms of increased intracranial pressure (ICP) is the nurse likely to determine in a 1-month-old infant? Select all that apply.

☐ **1.** Bulging fontanels

☐ **2.** Decreased blood pressure

☐ **3.** Increased pulse

☐ **4.** High-pitched cry

☐ **5.** Headache

☐ **6.** Irritability

Answer: 1, 4, 6

Rationale: Signs and symptoms of increased ICP in a 1-month-old include full, tense, bulging fontanels; a high-pitched cry; and irritability. With increased ICP, blood pressure rises while heart rate falls. The infant may have a headache, but the nurse is unable to ascertain this finding in an infant.

Nursing process step: Data collection

Client needs category: Physiological integrity

Client needs subcategory: Physiological adaptation

Cognitive level: Analysis

5. A nurse is checking a 10-month-old infant during a checkup. Which developmental milestones would the nurse expect the infant to display? Select all that apply.

☐ **1.** Holding head erect

☐ **2.** Self-feeding

☐ **3.** Demonstrating good bowel and bladder control

☐ **4.** Sitting on a firm surface without support

☐ **5.** Bearing majority of weight on legs

☐ **6.** Walking alone

Answer: 1, 4, 5

Rationale: By age 3 months, an infant should be able to hold his head erect. By age 10 months, he should be able to sit on a firm surface without support and bear the majority of his weight on his legs (for example, walking while holding on to furniture). Self-feeding and bowel and bladder control are developmental milestones of toddlers. By age 12 months, the infant should be able to stand alone and may take his first steps.

Nursing process step: Data collection

Client needs category: Health promotion and maintenance

Client needs subcategory: None

Cognitive level: Application

---

6. An 11-month-old is diagnosed with an ear infection—his second one. The mother asks why children experience more ear infections than adults. The nurse shows the mother a diagram of the ear and explains the differences in anatomy. Identify the portion of the infant's ear that allows fluid to stagnate and act as a medium for bacteria.

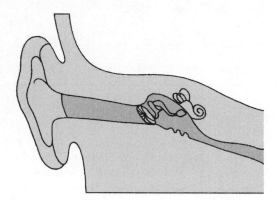

Answer:

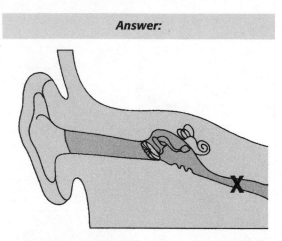

Rationale: The eustachian tube in an infant is shorter and wider than in an adult or an older child. It also slants horizontally. Because of these anatomic features, nasopharyngeal secretions can enter the middle ear more easily, stagnate, and tend to cause infections.

Nursing process step: Data collection

Client needs category: Health promotion and maintenance

Client needs subcategory: None

Cognitive level: Comprehension

7. A nurse is preparing to administer chloramphenicol (Chloromycetin Otic) to a 2-year-old with an infection of the external auditory canal. The order reads, "2 gtts A.D. t.i.d." Which steps should the nurse take to administer this medication? Select all that apply.

- ☐ **1.** Wash her hands and arrange supplies at the bedside.
- ☐ **2.** Warm the medication to body temperature.
- ☐ **3.** Lie the child on his right side with his left ear facing up.
- ☐ **4.** Examine the ear canal for drainage.
- ☐ **5.** Gently pull the pinna up and back and instill the drops into the external ear canal.

Answer: 1, 2, 4

Rationale: The nurse should prepare to instill the eardrops by washing her hands, gathering the supplies, and arranging the supplies at the bedside. To avoid adverse effects resulting from eardrops that are too cold (such as vertigo, nausea, and pain), the medication should be warmed to body temperature in a bowl of warm water. Temperature of the drops should be tested by placing a drop on the wrist. Before instilling the drops, the ear canal should be examined for drainage that may reduce the medication's effectiveness. Because the abbreviation "A.D." stands for "right ear," the child should be placed on his left side with his right ear facing up. For an infant or a child younger than age 3, gently pull the auricle down and back because the ear canal is straighter in children of this age-group.

Nursing process step: Implementation

Client needs category: Physiological integrity

Client needs subcategory: Pharmacological therapies

Cognitive level: Application

---

8. A nurse is teaching cardiopulmonary resuscitation (CPR) to the parents of a 1-month-old being discharged with an apnea monitor. Which steps are appropriate for performing CPR on an infant? Select all that apply.

- ☐ **1.** Open the airway by hyperextending the head.
- ☐ **2.** Pinch the nose before delivering a breath.
- ☐ **3.** Check for a pulse by palpating the brachial artery.
- ☐ **4.** Place the heel of one hand on the lower third of the sternum to perform compressions.
- ☐ **5.** Compress the sternum ½" to 1".
- ☐ **6.** Give five compressions to one breath.

Answer: 3, 5, 6

Rationale: When performing CPR on an infant, check for a brachial pulse by palpating the inside of the upper arm, midway between the elbow and shoulder. To provide compressions to an infant, compress the sternum ½" to 1" at a ratio of five compressions to one breath. Tilting the head too far back in an infant can block, rather than open, the airway. To deliver a breath to an infant, the rescuer should cover the infant's mouth and nose with her mouth. When performing chest compressions on an infant, the tips of the middle and ring fingers should be placed on the sternum, one finger's width below the nipple line.

Nursing process step: Implementation

Client needs category: Physiological integrity

Client needs subcategory: Reduction of risk potential

Cognitive level: Application

9. A nurse is providing preoperative teaching to the parents of a 9-month-old infant who's having surgery to repair a ventricular septal defect. Identify the area of the heart where the defect is located.

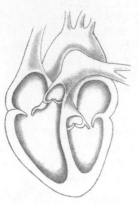

Answer:

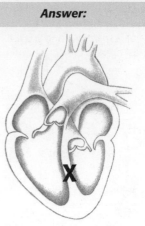

Rationale: A ventricular septal defect is a hole in the septum between the ventricles. The defect can be anywhere along the septum but is most commonly located in the middle of the septum.

Nursing process step: Implementation

Client needs category: Physiological integrity

Client needs subcategory: Physiological adaptation

Cognitive level: Comprehension

---

10. A nurse at the family clinic receives a call from the mother of a 5-week-old infant. The mother states that her child was diagnosed with colic at the last checkup. Unfortunately, the symptoms have remained the same. Which instructions are appropriate? Select all that apply.

☐ **1.** Position the infant on his back after feedings.

☐ **2.** Soothe the child by humming and rocking.

☐ **3.** Immediately bring the infant to the emergency department.

☐ **4.** Burp the infant adequately after feedings.

☐ **5.** Provide small but frequent feedings to the infant.

☐ **6.** Offer a pacifier if it isn't time for the infant to eat.

Answer: 2, 4, 5, 6

Rationale: Colic consists of recurrent paroxysmal bouts of abdominal pain and is fairly common in infants. It usually disappears by age 3 months. Rocking, riding in a car, humming, and offering a pacifier may be used to comfort the infant. Decreasing gas formation by frequent burping, giving smaller feedings more frequently, and positioning the infant in an upright seat are also appropriate teaching. The infant shouldn't be positioned on his back after feedings because this increases gas formation. Colic is a manageable condition in the home. The infant doesn't need to be taken to the emergency department unless the symptoms worsen, a temperature accompanies the symptoms, or vomiting occurs with the symptoms.

Nursing process step: Implementation

Client needs category: Physiological integrity

Client needs subcategory: Basic care and comfort

Cognitive level: Application

11. A 6-month-old is found floating face down in a swimming pool. A neighbor, who's a nurse, checks for the presence of respirations and a pulse. Identify the area that's most appropriate to check for a pulse.

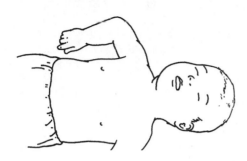

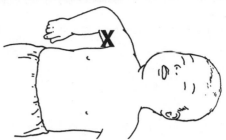

Rationale: An infant's pulse is most accessible at the brachial artery. The brachial artery is located inside the upper arm between the elbow and the shoulder. Cardiopulmonary resuscitation guidelines recommend using this area to check for a pulse.

Nursing process step: Data collection

Client needs category: Physiological integrity

Client needs subcategory: Physiological adaptation

Cognitive level: Application

---

12. A nurse is reviewing the teaching plan with the parents of an infant undergoing repair for a cleft lip. Which instructions should the nurse give? Select all that apply.

☐ **1.** Offer a pacifier as needed.

☐ **2.** Lay the infant on his back or side to sleep.

☐ **3.** Sit the infant up for each feeding.

☐ **4.** Loosen the arm restraints every 4 hours.

☐ **5.** Clean the suture line after each feeding by dabbing it with saline solution.

☐ **6.** Give the infant extra care and support.

Answer: 2, 3, 5, 6

Rationale: An infant with a repaired cleft lip should be put to sleep on his back or side to prevent trauma to the surgery site. He should be fed in the upright position with a syringe and attached tubing to prevent stress to the suture line from sucking. To prevent crusts and scarring, the suture line should be cleaned after each feeding by dabbing it with half-strength hydrogen peroxide or saline solution. The infant should receive extra care and support because he can't meet emotional needs by sucking. Extra care and support may also prevent crying, which stresses the suture line. Pacifiers shouldn't be used during the healing process because they stress the suture line. Arm restraints are used to keep the infant's hands away from the mouth and should be loosened every 2 hours.

Nursing process step: Implementation

Client needs category: Physiological integrity

Client needs subcategory: Reduction of risk potential

Cognitive level: Application

The toddler

1. A nurse is admitting a 14-month-old to the pediatric floor with diagnosis of croup. Which characteristics would the nurse expect the toddler to have if he's developing normally? Select all that apply.

☐ **1.** Strong hand grasp

☐ **2.** Tendency to hold one object while looking for another

☐ **3.** Recognition of familiar voices (smiles in recognition)

☐ **4.** Presence of Moro reflex

☐ **5.** Weight that is triple the birth weight

☐ **6.** Closed anterior fontanelle

Answer: 1, 2, 3, 5

Rationale: A strong hand grasp is demonstrated within the first month of life. Holding one object while looking for another is accomplished by the 20th week. Within the first year of life, the toddler masters smiling at familiar faces and voices, the Moro reflex disappears, and birth weight triples. The anterior fontanel closes at approximately age 18 months.

Nursing process step: Data collection

Client needs category: Health promotion and maintenance

Client needs subcategory: None

Cognitive level: Application

2. A 13-month-old is admitted to the pediatric unit with a diagnosis of gastroenteritis. The toddler has experienced vomiting and diarrhea for the past 3 days, and laboratory tests reveal that he's dehydrated. Which nursing interventions are correct to prevent further dehydration? Select all that apply.

☐ **1.** Encourage the child to eat a balanced diet.

☐ **2.** Give clear liquids in small amounts.

☐ **3.** Give milk in small amounts.

☐ **4.** Encourage the child to eat nonsalty soups and broths.

☐ **5.** Monitor the I.V. solution per the physician's order.

☐ **6.** Withhold all solid food and liquids until the symptoms pass.

Answer: 2, 4, 5

Rationale: A child experiencing nausea and vomiting would not be able to tolerate a regular diet. He should be given sips of clear liquids, and the diet should be advanced as tolerated. Unsalty soups and broths are appropriate clear liquids. Milk should not be given because it can worsen the child's diarrhea. I.V. fluids should be monitored to maintain the fluid status and help to rehydrate the child. Solid foods may be withheld throughout the acute phase; however, clear fluids should be encouraged in small amounts (3 to 4 tablespoons every half hour).

Nursing process step: Implementation

Client needs category: Physiological integrity

Client needs subcategory: Basic care and comfort

Cognitive level: Application

3. An acutely ill, 20-month-old toddler is admitted to the hospital with sickle cell crisis. The child is crying, restless, and appears uncomfortable when touched. Vital signs show slightly elevated heart rate and blood pressure and a temperature of 102°F (38.8°C). Which nursing diagnoses would a nurse expect to see included in the care plan? Select all that apply.

☐ **1.** *Ineffective airway clearance*

☐ **2.** *Acute pain*

☐ **3.** *Unbalanced nutrition*

☐ **4.** *Risk for infection*

☐ **5.** *Powerlessness*

☐ **6.** *Risk for impaired parent/child attachment*

Answer: 2, 4

Rationale: In a vaso-occlusive crisis, sickle-shaped cells stick and clump together, obstructing normal blood flow. A thrombus may form and obstruct circulation, possibly leading to tissue death. Severe pain in the affected body parts is the characteristic symptom when tissue is denied normal blood circulation. The child has an elevated temperature. Although there's no other evidence presented of current infection, clients in a crisis are more prone to infection, so a risk of infection diagnosis is appropriate. There's no evidence presented of ineffective airway clearance, unbalanced nutrition, powerlessness, or impaired family/child attachment issues.

Nursing process step: Planning

Client needs category: Physiological integrity

Client needs subcategory: Basic care and comfort

Cognitive level: Analysis

√

4. A toddler is ordered 350 mg of amoxicillin (Augmentin) by mouth four times per day. The pharmacy sends a bottle of amoxicillin with a concentration of 250 mg/5 ml. How many milliliters should the nurse administer per dose?

_____

Answer: 7

Rationale: The following formula is used to calculate drug dosages:

Dose on hand/Quantity on hand = Dose desired/X

In this example, the equation is as follows:

$$250 \text{ mg}/5 \text{ ml} = 350 \text{ mg}/X$$

$$X = 7 \text{ ml.}$$

Nursing process step: Implementation

Client needs category: Physiological integrity

Client needs subcategory: Pharmacological therapies

Cognitive level: Application

5. A 3-year-old is admitted to the pediatric unit with pneumonia. He has a productive cough and appears to have difficulty breathing. The parents tell the nurse that the toddler hasn't been eating or drinking much and has been very inactive. Which interventions to improve airway clearance should the nurse expect in the care plan? Select all that apply.

☐ **1.** Restrict fluid intake.

☐ **2.** Perform chest physiotherapy as ordered.

☐ **3.** Encourage coughing and deep breathing.

☐ **4.** Keep the head of the bed flat.

☐ **5.** Perform postural drainage.

☐ **6.** Maintain humidification with a cool mist humidifier.

Answer: 2, 3, 5, 6

Rationale: Chest physiotherapy and postural drainage work together to break up congestion and then drain secretions. Coughing and deep breathing are also effective to remove congestion. A cool mist humidifier helps loosen thick mucus and relax airway passages. Fluids should be encouraged—not restricted. The child should be placed in semi-Fowler's or high Fowler's position to facilitate breathing and promote optimal lung expansion.

Nursing process step: Planning

Client needs category: Physiological integrity

Client needs subcategory: Basic care and comfort

Cognitive level: Application

The preschooler

1. A nurse is observing the parents of a 4-year-old who has been admitted to the hospital. Which actions indicate that the parents understand how to best minimize anxiety during their child's hospitalization? Select all that apply.

☐ **1.** The parents bring the child's favorite toy to the hospital.

☐ **2.** The parents explain all procedures to the child in great detail.

☐ **3.** The parents remain at the child's side during the hospitalization.

☐ **4.** The parents bring the child's siblings for a brief visit.

☐ **5.** The parents leave the room when the child undergoes a painful procedure.

☐ **6.** The parents punish the child if the child isn't cooperative.

Answer: 1, 3, 4

Rationale: The most effective means of minimizing the child's anxiety during hospitalization is to have the parents stay with him. Having a familiar toy helps the child to deal with the anxiety of unfamiliar surroundings. Sibling visitation can also help to ease the child's anxiety. Explaining a procedure to a young child in great detail only maximizes fear. Parents can be effective in calming and comforting a child during painful procedures, so they should remain in the room. Rewards, not punishment, should be offered to a preschooler.

Nursing process step: Evaluation

Client needs category: Psychosocial integrity

Client needs subcategory: None

Cognitive level: Analysis

2. A 5-year-old preschooler suspected of having leukemia is admitted to the hospital for diagnosis and treatment. A bone marrow aspiration is ordered. Place the interventions below in ascending chronological order as to how the nurse should perform them, based on importance. Use all the options.

1. Give the child his own biopsy kit: a syringe without a needle, cotton balls, and adhesive bandages, and act out the procedure by using a doll or stuffed animal.

2. Reassure him that the pain will go away quickly.

3. Check the biopsy site for bleeding and inflammation and observe the child for signs and symptoms of hemorrhage and infection.

4. Discuss the procedure with his parents and the plan for preparing the child.

5. Explain the kinds of pressure and discomfort he'll feel during the procedure and that it's OK to cry.

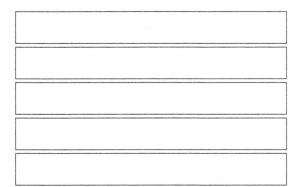

Answer:

4. Discuss the procedure with his parents and the plan for preparing the child.

1. Give the child his own biopsy kit: a syringe without a needle, cotton balls, and adhesive bandages, and act out the procedure by using a doll or stuffed animal.

5. Explain the kinds of pressure and discomfort he'll feel during the procedure and that it's OK to cry.

2. Reassure him that the pain will go away quickly.

3. Check the biopsy site for bleeding and inflammation and observe the child for signs and symptoms of hemorrhage and infection.

Rationale: The nurse must first discuss the procedure with the parents and encourage them to get involved with the plan for preparing the child. Next the nurse should use play to teach the child about the procedure to help gain the child's confidence and put the child at ease. After the child is comfortable, the nurse can explain the discomfort he'll feel and then reassure him that the pain will go away. Lastly, postprocedure the nurse needs to check for bleeding, inflammation, and signs and symptoms of pain and infection.

Nursing process step: Planning

Client needs category: Physiological integrity

Client needs subcategory: Physiological adaptation

Cognitive level: Analysis

---

3. A preschooler is in danger of becoming dehydrated as a result of vomiting and diarrhea. The nurse realizes that dehydration can be prevented if intake is sufficient to produce a urine output of 3 ml/kg/hr. The preschooler weighs 44 lb. What is the minimum urine output in milliliters that should be achieved in an 8-hour shift in order to prevent dehydration?

Answer: 480

Rationale: First, convert the child's weight from pounds to kilograms. There are 2.2 kg in 1 lb.

$$44 \div 2.2 = 20$$

$$3 \text{ ml} \times 20 \text{ kg} \times 8 \text{ hours} = 480 \text{ ml.}$$

Nursing process step: Data collection

Client needs category: Physiological integrity

Client needs subcategory: Reduction of risk potential

Cognitive level: Comprehension

4. A preschooler is being admitted to the hospital and isolation precautions need to be implemented. Based on the progress note below, which isolation precautions would be used for this client?

11/8/06	5-year-old with varicella admitted with high
1100	fever, dehydration, and pruritic rash on
	face and trunk with lesions in all stages. See
	graphic record for vital signs. I.V. started
	in ℚ arm. Isolation precautions instituted.
	———————————— J. Trump, RN

☐ **1.** Standard precautions

☐ **2.** Airborne precautions

☐ **3.** Droplet precautions

☐ **4.** Contact precautions

Answer: 2

Rationale: Airborne precautions are appropriate because varicella is transmitted by airborne droplet nuclei of small particles that can be dispersed by air currents within a room. Standard precautions are used for all clients regardless of diagnosis and alone would not be appropriate for the client with varicella. Droplet precautions are used for illness transmitted by large-particle droplets that can be spread by coughing, sneezing, and talking, such as influenza, mumps, and diphtheria. Contact precautions are used for a client with an illness spread by direct client contact or by contact with items in the client's environment, such as GI, respiratory, or skin or wound infections.

Nursing process step: Implementation

Client needs category: Safe, effective care environment

Client needs subcategory: Safety and infection control

Cognitive level: Application

---

5. A nurse is caring for a 4-year-old who's in the terminal stages of cancer. Which statements are true? Select all that apply.

☐ **1.** The parents may be at different stages in dealing with the child's death.

☐ **2.** The child is thinking about the future and knows he may not be able to participate.

☐ **3.** The dying child may become clingy and act like a toddler.

☐ **4.** Whispering in the child's room will help the child to cope.

☐ **5.** The death of a child may have long-term disruptive effects on the family.

☐ **6.** The child doesn't fully understand the concept of death.

Answer: 1, 3, 5, 6

Rationale: When dealing with a dying child, parents may be at different stages of grief at different times. The child may regress in his behaviors. The stress of a child's death often results in divorce and behavioral problems in siblings. Preschoolers see illness and death as a form of punishment. Preschoolers fear separation from their parents and may worry about who will provide care for them after death. Thinking about the future is typical of an adolescent facing death, not a preschooler, though preschoolers have a rudimentary concept of time. Whispering in front of the child only increases his fear.

Nursing process step: Planning

Client needs category: Psychosocial integrity

Client needs subcategory: None

Cognitive level: Analysis

---

6. A 5-year-old is brought to the emergency department after being given aspirin for many days for flulike symptoms; he's diagnosed with Reye's syndrome. The client has progressed to stage III of the syndrome. A nurse is preparing for the next stages of the syndrome and knows that the syndrome develops in five stages. Place the stages listed below in ascending chronological order. Use all the options.

1. Brief recovery period: child doesn't seem ill

2. Coma

3. Viral infection

4. Deep coma, seizures, decreased tendon reflexes, and respiratory failure

5. Intractable vomiting; lethargy; rapidly changing mental status; increasing blood pressure, respiratory, and pulse rate; hyperactive reflexes

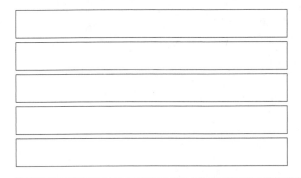

Answer:

3. Viral infection

1. Brief recovery period: child doesn't seem ill

5. Intractable vomiting; lethargy; rapidly changing mental status; increasing blood pressure, respiratory, and pulse rate; hyperactive reflexes

2. Coma

4. Deep coma, seizures, decreased tendon reflexes, and respiratory failure

Rationale: Administration of aspirin during a viral illness has been implicated as a contributing factor in Reye's syndrome. The order listed is the order in which the syndrome develops, with the third stage when the syndrome is commonly diagnosed.

Nursing process step: Planning

Client needs category: Physiological integrity

Client needs subcategory: Physiological adaptation

Cognitive level: Analysis

---

7. A school nurse is conducting registration for a first grader. Which immunizations should the school nurse verify the child has had on entering school? Select all that apply.

☐ **1.** Hepatitis B series

☐ **2.** Diphtheria-tetanus-pertussis series

☐ **3.** *Haemophilus influenzae* type b series

☐ **4.** Varicella zoster

☐ **5.** Pneumonia vaccine

☐ **6.** Oral polio series

Answer: 1, 2, 3

Rationale: Hepatitis B series, diphtheria-tetanus-pertussis series, *H. influenzae* type b series, and inactivated, not oral, polio series are immunizations that the child should receive before entering first grade. The oral polio vaccine was discontinued in 1999 for the safer inactivated polio vaccine (IPV). The varicella zoster vaccine is administered only if the child hasn't had chickenpox. Pneumonia vaccine isn't required or routinely given to children.

Nursing process step: Data collection

Client needs category: Health promotion and maintenance

Client needs subcategory: None

Cognitive level: Knowledge

8. A preschooler is diagnosed with a right Wilms' tumor and the nurse is preparing teaching material for the family. On this drawing of the urinary system, which area would a nurse identify as that in which the tumor can be found?

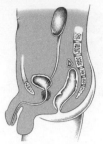

Answer:

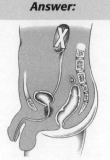

Rationale: Wilms' tumor, also called *nephroblastoma,* is located in the kidney. It's the most common intra-abdominal tumor in children ages 2 to 4, and favors the left kidney.

Nursing process step: Data collection

Client needs category: Physiological integrity

Client needs subcategory: Physiological adaptation

Cognitive level: Application

The school-age child

1. A nurse in a pediatrician's office is determining the cognitive ability of a 7-year-old child who's in first grade. Using a block test, the child demonstrates an understanding of conservation of mass. The nurse, who's knowledgeable in Piaget's theory of cognitive development, knows the child is in the concrete operational stage of Piaget's stages. Place the stages listed below in ascending chronological order. Use all the options.

| 1. Concrete operational stage |
| 2. Sensorimotor stage |
| 3. Preoperational stage |
| 4. Formal operational thought stage |

| |
| |
| |
| |

Answer:

| 2. Sensorimotor stage |
| 3. Preoperational stage |
| 1. Concrete operational stage |
| 4. Formal operational thought stage |

Rationale: The sensorimotor stage is characterized by an understanding of object permanence, causality, and spatial relationships. The preoperational stage is marked by egocentricity, mastering representational language and symbols, and transudative reasoning. In the concrete operational stage, the child masters sorting, ordering, and classifying facts to use in problem solving. In the formal operational thought stage, the child masters abstract ideas, possibilities, inductive reasoning, and complex deductive reasoning.

Nursing process step: Evaluation

Client needs category: Health promotion and maintenance

Client needs subcategory: None

Cognitive level: Analysis

2. An 11-year-old child is brought to the emergency department from a soccer game, complaining of difficulty breathing. The mother states that this has occurred a few times during recent soccer games, although not as severely as the current episode. The client has rapid, labored breathing with expiratory wheezes and a temperature of 98.8° F (37.1° C). A nurse assists with care based on a nursing diagnosis of which symptoms? Select all that apply.

☐ **1.** *Activity intolerance related to exertional asthma*

☐ **2.** *Ineffective breathing pattern related to pneumonia*

☐ **3.** *Risk for infection related to possible tuberculosis (TB)*

☐ **4.** *Impaired gas exchange related to pulmonary embolus*

☐ **5.** *Ineffective airway clearance related to croup*

Answer: 1

Rationale: *Activity intolerance related to exertional asthma* is the correct response because asthma is a chronic inflammatory airway disorder that causes episodic airway obstruction and hyperresponsiveness of the airway to multiple stimuli. Asthma is characterized by wheezing, shortness of breath, exercise intolerance, reduced expiratory flow, recurrent cough, and respiratory distress. A client with pneumonia would present with an elevated temperature, rhonchi, crackles, wheezing, dyspnea, tachypnea, and restlessness. TB signs and symptoms would include chronic cough, anorexia and weight loss, and fever. Symptoms of pulmonary embolism include dyspnea on exertion, tachycardia, elevated blood pressure, dependent crackles, and a cough with frothy, blood-tinged sputum, progressing to cardiogenic shock. Croup affects younger children (younger than age 5 years) and is characterized by a barking cough, inspiratory stridor, pallor, restlessness, low-grade fever, crackles, rhonchi, and expiratory wheezing with worsening symptoms at night.

Nursing process step: Implementation

Client needs category: Physiological integrity

Client needs subcategory: Physiological adaptation

Cognitive level: Analysis

---

3. An 11-year-old boy is brought to a rural clinic listless and pale. The parents state that the child had a "bad sore throat" 2 weeks ago and that they had him gargle with salt water. The parents report that they saw improvement but now the child has flulike symptoms. The child is diagnosed with rheumatic fever. Which signs and symptoms are associated with rheumatic fever? Select all that apply.

☐ **1.** Nausea and vomiting

☐ **2.** Polyarthritis

☐ **3.** Chorea

☐ **4.** High-grade fever

☐ **5.** Carditis

☐ **6.** Rash

Answer: 2, 3, 5, 6

Rationale: Characteristic manifestations of rheumatic fever include polyarthritis, chorea, carditis, and a red rash. The child doesn't usually experience nausea and vomiting. He may have a minor low-grade fever in the afternoon.

Nursing process step: Data collection

Client needs category: Physiological integrity

Client needs subcategory: Physiological adaptation

Cognitive level: Application

4. A 9-year-old boy with diabetes tests his glucose level before lunch in the nurse's office. According to his sliding scale of insulin, he's due for 1 unit of regular insulin. What steps should a nurse follow after confirming the medication order, washing her hands, drawing up the appropriate dose, verifying the boy's identity, and putting on gloves? Put the following steps in ascending chronological order. Use all the options.

1.	Pinch the skin around the injection site.

2.	Release the skin and give the injection.

3.	Clean the injection site with alcohol and loosen the needle cover.

4.	Select an appropriate injection site, being sure to discuss with the client so the sites are rotated.

5.	Cover the site with an alcohol pad. Press but don't rub the site.

6.	Uncover the needle; insert it at a 45- to 90-degree angle.

4.	Select an appropriate injection site, being sure to discuss with the client so the sites are rotated.

3.	Clean the injection site with alcohol and loosen the needle cover.

1.	Pinch the skin around the injection site.

6.	Uncover the needle; insert it at a 45- to 90-degree angle.

2.	Release the skin and give the injection.

5.	Cover the site with an alcohol pad. Press but don't rub the site.

Rationale: The above order shows the appropriate steps for giving a subcutaneous insulin injection.

Nursing process step: Implementation

Client needs category: Physiological integrity

Client needs subcategory: Pharmacological therapies

Cognitive level: Application

---

5. When talking with 10- and 11-year-old children about death, the nurse should incorporate which guidelines? Select all that apply.

☐ **1.** Logical explanations aren't appropriate.

☐ **2.** The children will be curious about the physical aspects of death.

☐ **3.** The children will know that death is inevitable and irreversible.

☐ **4.** The children will be influenced by the attitudes of the adults in their lives.

Rationale: By age 9 or 10, most children know that death is universal, inevitable, and irreversible. School-age children are curious about the physical aspects of death and may wonder what happens to the body. Their cognitive abilities are advanced and they respond well to logical explanations. The adults in their environment influence their attitudes towards death. Adults should be encouraged to include children in family rituals.

Nursing process step: Implementation

Client needs category: Psychosocial integrity

Client needs subcategory: None

Cognitive level: Application

6. A 7-year-old client is admitted to the hospital for treatment of facial cellulitis. He's admitted for observation and for administration of a 10-day course of I.V. antibiotics. Which interventions would help this client cope with the insertion of a peripheral I.V. line? Select all that apply.

☐ **1.** Explain the procedure to the child immediately before the procedure.

☐ **2.** Apply a topical anesthetic to the I.V. site before the procedure.

☐ **3.** Ask the child which hand he uses for drawing.

☐ **4.** Explain the procedure to the child using abstract terms.

☐ **5.** Don't let the child see the equipment to be used in the procedure.

☐ **6.** Tell the child that the procedure won't hurt.

Answer: 2, 3

Rationale: Topical anesthetics reduce the pain of a venipuncture. Asking which hand the child draws with helps to identify the dominant hand. The I.V. should be inserted into the opposite extremity so that the child can continue his usual activities with little disruption. Younger school-age children don't have the capability for abstract thinking. The procedure should be explained using simple words. The child should have the procedure explained to him well before it takes place so that he has time to ask questions. There's usually some pain or discomfort involved in venipuncture despite anesthetics, so the child shouldn't be told otherwise.

Nursing process step: Implementation

Client needs category: Psychosocial integrity

Client needs subcategory: None

Cognitive level: Application

---

7. When teaching bicycle safety to children and parents, a nurse should stress protecting which part of the body?

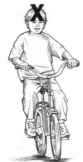

Answer:

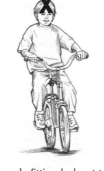

Rationale: A properly fitting helmet to protect the head is the most important safety feature to stress to children and parents.

Nursing process step: Implementation

Client needs category: Physiological integrity

Client needs subcategory: Reduction of risk potential

Cognitive level: Application

8. A 6-year-old girl is brought to the pediatrician's office by her mother for evaluation. The child recently started wetting the bed and running a low-grade fever. A urinalysis is positive for bacteria and protein. A diagnosis of a urinary tract infection (UTI) is made and the child is prescribed antibiotics. Which interventions are appropriate? Select all that apply.

☐ **1.** Limit fluids for the next few days to decrease the frequency of urination.

☐ **2.** Assess the mother's understanding of UTIs and its causes.

☐ **3.** Instruct the mother to administer the antibiotic as prescribed — even if the symptoms diminish.

☐ **4.** Provide instructions only to the mother, not the child.

☐ **5.** Discourage the use of bubble bath.

☐ **6.** Tell the mother to have the child wipe from the back to the front after voiding and defecation.

Answer: 2, 3, 5

Rationale: Assessing the mother's understanding of UTI and its causes provides the nurse with a baseline for teaching. The full course of antibiotics must be given to eradicate the organism and prevent recurrence, even if the child's signs and symptoms decrease. Bubble bath can irritate the vulva and urethra and contribute to the development of a UTI. Fluids should be encouraged, not limited, in order to prevent urinary stasis and help flush the organism out of the urinary tract. Instructions should be given to the child at her level of understanding to help her better understand the treatment and promote compliance. The child should wipe from the front to the back, not back to front, to minimize the risk of contamination after elimination.

Nursing process step: Implementation

Client needs category: Health promotion and maintenance

Client needs subcategory: None

Cognitive level: Application

The adolescent

1. Which symptoms reported by an adolescent's parents indicate that the adolescent is abusing amphetamines? Select all that apply.

☐ **1.** Restlessness

☐ **2.** Fatigue

☐ **3.** Talkativeness

☐ **4.** Excessive perspiration

☐ **5.** Watery eyes

☐ **6.** Excessive nasal drainage

Answer: 1, 3, 4

Rationale: Amphetamines are central nervous system stimulants. Symptoms of amphetamine abuse include marked nervousness, restlessness, excitability, talkativeness, and excessive perspiration.

Nursing process step: Data collection

Client needs category: Health promotion and maintenance

Client needs subcategory: None

Cognitive level: Application

2. A group of 16-year-olds are eating at a restaurant. One adolescent starts to cough then can't get a breath. He puts his hands around his neck to gesture that he can't breathe. A friend stands and positions himself to begin the Heimlich maneuver. Identify the area where it's most appropriate to place the hands when performing the Heimlich maneuver.

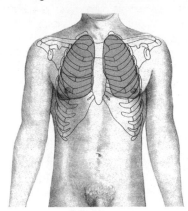

Answer:

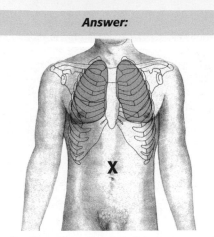

Rationale: To perform the Heimlich maneuver, the rescuer should place his hands on the abdomen, just above the navel.

Nursing process step: Implementation

Client needs category: Physiological integrity

Client needs subcategory: Physiological adaptation

Cognitive level: Application

---

3. A 15-year-old boy is admitted to the telemetry unit because of a suspected cardiac arrhythmia. The nurse applies five electrodes to his chest and attaches the leadwires. Identify the area where she would place the chest lead (V_1).

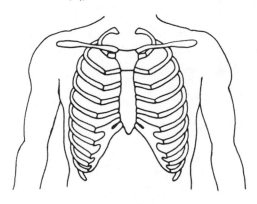

Answer:

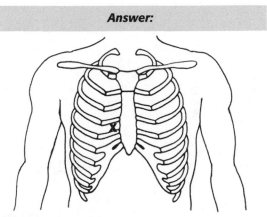

Rationale: The V_1 lead is placed in the 4th intercostal space to the right of the sternum.

Nursing process step: Data collection

Client needs category: Physiological integrity

Client needs subcategory: Reduction of risk potential

Cognitive level: Knowledge

4. A 14-year-old diagnosed with acne vulgaris asks what causes it. Which factors should the nurse identify for this client? Select all that apply.

☐ **1.** Chocolates and sweets

☐ **2.** Increased hormone levels

☐ **3.** Growth of anaerobic bacteria

☐ **4.** Caffeine

☐ **5.** Heredity

☐ **6.** Fatty foods

Answer: 2, 3, 5

Rationale: Acne vulgaris is characterized by the appearance of comedones (blackheads and whiteheads). Comedones develop for various reasons, including increased hormone levels, growth of anaerobic bacteria, heredity, and irritation or application of irritating substances (such as cosmetics). A direct relationship between acne vulgaris and consumption of chocolates, caffeine, or fatty foods hasn't been established.

Nursing process step: Implementation

Client needs category: Physiological integrity

Client needs subcategory: Physiological adaptation

Cognitive level: Application

---

5. A 16-year-old with diabetes is ordered to receive 15 units of NPH insulin and 5 units of regular insulin. Both are dispensed from the pharmacy in 100 units/ml vials. How many total ml should the nurse administer?

_____

Answer: 0.2

Rationale: Use the following equation:

$$100 \text{ units/ml} = 15 \text{ units}/X$$

$$X = 0.15 \text{ ml.}$$

$$100 \text{ units/ml} = 5 \text{ units}/X$$

$$X = 0.05 \text{ ml.}$$

Add to get the total sum: $0.15 + 0.05 = 0.2$ ml.

Nursing process step: Implementation

Client needs category: Physiological integrity

Client needs subcategory: Pharmacological therapies

Cognitive level: Application

6. A 13-year-old with cystic fibrosis is admitted to the hospital with a pulmonary infection. A physician orders 2 mg/kg of an oral solution of prednisone daily to be divided into 4 doses. The oral solution has 5 mg/ml and the child weighs 99 lb. How many ml should the nurse administer for one dose?

(2.5mL)

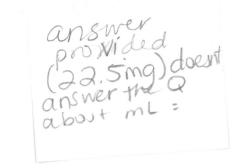
answer provided (22.5mg) doesnt answer the Q about mL =

Answer: 22.5

Rationale: The nurse should first convert the child's weight to kilograms.

Use this equation, cross multiply, and solve for X.

$$1 \text{ kg}/2.2 \text{ lb} = X \text{ kg}/99 \text{ lb}$$

$$2.2X = 99$$

$$X = 45 \text{ kg.}$$

Then, calculate the daily dosage by using this formula:

$$45 \text{ kg} \times 2 \text{ mg/kg} = 90 \text{ mg.}$$

To calculate the amount of each dosage, divide by 4:

$$90 \text{ mg}/4 = 22.5 \text{ mg.}$$

Nursing process step: Implementation

Client needs category: Physiological integrity

Client needs subcategory: Pharmacological therapies

Cognitive level: Application

---

7. A nurse is reviewing teaching points with an adolescent with inflammatory bowel disease. The topic is the use of corticosteroids. Which adverse effects are concerns for this client? Select all that apply.

☐ **1.** Acne

☐ **2.** Hirsutism

☐ **3.** Mood swings

☐ **4.** Osteoporosis

☐ **5.** Growth spurts

☐ **6.** Adrenal suppression

Answer: 1, 2, 3, 4, 6

Rationale: Adverse effects of corticosteroids include acne, hirsutism, mood swings, osteoporosis, and adrenal suppression. Steroid use in children and adolescents may cause delayed growth, not growth spurts.

Nursing process step: Implementation

Client needs category: Physiological integrity

Client needs subcategory: Pharmacological therapies

Cognitive level: Application

Psychiatric and mental health nursing

Foundations of psychiatric nursing

1. Knowledge of Maslow's hierarchy of needs can assist a nurse in understanding client behavior. Place the stages of Maslow's hierarchy of needs in order from basic to most complex. Use all the options.

1. Safety and security
2. Self-esteem
3. Physiologic needs
4. Love and belonging
5. Self-actualization

Answer:

3. Physiologic needs
1. Safety and security
4. Love and belonging
2. Self-esteem
5. Self-actualization

Rationale: Maslow's hierarchy of needs progresses from the most basic to the most complex needs. Maslow's theory states that physiologic needs are the most basic human needs. Only after physiologic needs have been met can safety concerns be addressed followed by love and belonging, which then fosters self-esteem and finally self-actualization.

Nursing process step: Planning

Client needs category: Psychosocial integrity

Client needs subcategory: None

Cognitive level: Application

2. Electroconvulsive therapy (ECT) is an effective treatment for severe depression when which conditions accompany it? Select all that apply.

☐ **1.** The client also has dementia.

☐ **2.** The client can't tolerate tricyclic antidepressants.

☐ **3.** The client lives in a long-term care facility.

☐ **4.** The client is undergoing a stressful life change.

☐ **5.** The client is having acute suicidal thoughts.

☐ **6.** The client is severely depressed despite taking numerous antidepressants.

Answer: 2, 5, 6

Rationale: ECT is used to treat acute depressive illnesses in an attempt to rapidly reverse a life-threatening situation, such as disturbing delusions, agitation, or suicide. ECT is also used when multiple antidepressants have been used but remain ineffective. New antidepressants may take weeks to become effective. The decision to use ECT isn't based on where the client lives. ECT isn't usually indicated for situational depressions or in those clients with dementia.

Nursing process step: Planning

Client needs category: Psychosocial integrity

Client needs subcategory: None

Cognitive level: Application

3. Characteristics of a therapeutic relationship are exemplified by meeting which goals? Select all that apply.

☐ **1.** The needs of the client and nurse are identified and met.

☐ **2.** The nurse helps the client explore different problem-solving techniques.

☐ **3.** The nurse encourages the practice of new coping skills.

☐ **4.** The nurse gives advice to the client.

☐ **5.** The nurse and client exchange personal information.

☐ **6.** The nurse discusses the client's feelings with family members.

Answer: 2, 3

Rationale: The goal of a therapeutic relationship is to enhance the personal growth of the client. Giving advice, exchanging personal information, and striving to meet the personal needs of the nurse and the client aren't therapeutic for the client and cross the boundaries of professionalism. Discussing information from or about the client with family members is a breach of confidentiality unless the client has expressly requested that the information be disclosed.

Nursing process step: Implementation

Client needs category: Psychosocial integrity

Client needs subcategory: None

Cognitive level: Analysis

---

4. A nurse understands that the first step in caring for a client with a mental health illness is to establish a therapeutic relationship to achieve effective communication. Place the phases of a therapeutic relationship in ascending chronological order. Use all the options.

| **1.** Working phase |
| **2.** Preinteraction phase |
| **3.** Termination phase |
| **4.** Orientation phase |

| |
| |
| |
| |

Answer:

| **2.** Preinteraction phase |
| **4.** Orientation phase |
| **1.** Working phase |
| **3.** Termination phase |

Rationale: The preinteraction phase in the initial phase includes the evaluation of the client by the nurse; the client is not often involved in this phase. The orientation phase is the "getting-to-know-you" phase in which trust begins to develop. The working phase involves participation by the nurse and client. The final phase is the termination phase, during which time the nurse and client evaluate the goals achieved or not achieved.

Nursing process step: Planning

Client needs category: Psychosocial integrity

Client needs subcategory: None

Cognitive level: Application

---

5. A nurse is explaining the Bill of Rights for psychiatric clients to a client who has voluntarily sought admission to an inpatient psychiatric facility. Which rights should the nurse include in the discussion? Select all that apply.

☐ **1.** Right to select health care team members

☐ **2.** Right to refuse treatment

☐ **3.** Right to a written treatment plan

☐ **4.** Right to obtain disability

☐ **5.** Right to confidentiality

☐ **6.** Right to personal mail

Answer: 2, 3, 5, 6

Rationale: An inpatient client usually receives a copy of the Bill of Rights for psychiatric patients, which includes the right to refuse treatment, the right to a written treatment plan, the right to confidentiality, and the right to personal mail. However, a client in an inpatient setting cannot select health team members. A client may apply for disability as a result of a chronic, incapacitating illness; however, disability is not a patient right, and members of a psychiatric institution do not decide who should receive it.

Nursing process step: Implementation

Client needs category: Psychosocial integrity

Client needs subcategory: None

Cognitive level: Application

---

6. In the emergency department, a client reveals to the nurse a lethal plan for committing suicide and agrees to a voluntary admission to the psychiatric unit. Which information will the nurse discuss with the client to answer the question, "How long do I have to stay here?" Select all that apply.

☐ **1.** "You may leave the hospital at any time unless you are suicidal, homicidal, or unable to meet basic needs."

☐ **2.** "Let's talk more after the health team has assessed you."

☐ **3.** "Once you've signed the papers, you have no say."

☐ **4.** "Because you could hurt yourself, you must be safe before being discharged."

☐ **5.** "You need a lawyer to help you make that decision."

☐ **6.** "There must be a court hearing before you leave the hospital."

Answer: 1, 2, 4

Rationale: A person who's admitted to a psychiatric hospital on a voluntary basis may sign out of the hospital unless the health care team determines that the person is harmful to himself or others. The health care team evaluates the client's condition before discharge. If there's reason to believe that the client is harmful to himself or others, a hearing can be held to determine if the admission status should be changed from voluntary to involuntary. Saying the client has no say once papers are signed is incorrect because it denies the client's rights. The client doesn't need a lawyer to leave the hospital. A hearing isn't mandated before discharge; a hearing is held only if the client remains unsafe and requires further treatment.

Nursing process step: Implementation

Client needs category: Psychosocial integrity

Client needs subcategory: None

Cognitive level: Application

7. A nurse has developed a relationship with a client who has an addiction problem. Which information would indicate that the therapeutic interaction is in the working stage? Select all that apply.

- ☐ **1.** The client addresses how the addiction has contributed to family distress.
- ☐ **2.** The client reluctantly shares the family history of addiction.
- ☐ **3.** The client verbalizes difficulty identifying personal strengths.
- ☐ **4.** The client discusses the financial problems related to the addiction.
- ☐ **5.** The client expresses uncertainty about meeting with the nurse.
- ☐ **6.** The client acknowledges the addiction's effects on the children.

Answer: 1, 3, 6

Rationale: In the working phase, the client explores, evaluates, and determines solutions to identified problems. Sharing a family history of addiction, discussing financial problems due to addiction, and expressing uncertainty about meeting the nurse would occur during the introductory phase of the nurse-client interaction.

Nursing process step: Evaluation

Client needs category: Psychosocial integrity

Client needs subcategory: None

Cognitive level: Application

Anxiety disorders

1. After receiving a referral from the occupational health nurse, a client comes to the mental health clinic with a suspected diagnosis of obsessive-compulsive disorder. The client explains that his compulsion to wash his hands is interfering with his job. Which interventions are appropriate when caring for a client with this disorder? Select all that apply.

- ☐ **1.** Don't allow the client time to carry out the ritualistic behavior.
- ☐ **2.** Support the use of appropriate defense mechanisms.
- ☐ **3.** Encourage the client to suppress his anxious feelings.
- ☐ **4.** Explore the patterns leading to the compulsive behavior.
- ☐ **5.** Listen attentively, but don't offer feedback.
- ☐ **6.** Encourage activities such as listening to music.

Answer: 2, 4, 6

Rationale: Client care should focus on reducing associated anxiety, fear, and guilt. The client should be encouraged to use appropriate defense mechanisms and express his feelings of anxiety. Exploring patterns that lead to the compulsive behavior may also be effective. Activities such as listening to music may divert the client's attention from unwanted thoughts. The client should be allowed to carry out ritualistic behavior until he can be distracted to some other activity. The nurse should always listen attentively to the client and offer feedback.

Nursing process step: Implementation

Client needs category: Psychosocial integrity

Client needs subcategory: None

Cognitive level: Application

2. After being examined by the forensic nurse in the emergency department, a rape victim is prepared for discharge. Due to the nature of the attack, this client is at risk for posttraumatic stress disorder (PTSD). Which symptoms are associated with PTSD? Select all that apply.

☐ **1.** Recurrent, intrusive recollections or nightmares

☐ **2.** Gingival and dental problems

☐ **3.** Sleep disturbances

☐ **4.** Flight of ideas

☐ **5.** Unusual talkativeness

☐ **6.** Difficulty concentrating

Answer: 1, 3, 6

Rationale: Clients diagnosed with PTSD typically experience recurrent, intrusive recollections or nightmares, sleep disturbances, difficulty concentrating, chronic anxiety or panic attacks, memory impairment, and feelings of detachment or estrangement that destroy interpersonal relationships. Gingival and dental problems are associated with bulimia. Flight of ideas and unusual talkativeness are characteristic of the acute manic phase of bipolar affective disorder.

Nursing process step: Data collection

Client needs category: Psychosocial integrity

Client needs subcategory: None

Cognitive level: Comprehension

3. A physician prescribes clomipramine (Anafranil) for a client diagnosed with obsessive-compulsive disorder. What instructions should the nurse include when teaching the client about this medication? Select all that apply.

☐ **1.** Avoid hazardous activities that require alertness or good coordination until adverse central nervous system (CNS) effects are known.

☐ **2.** Avoid alcohol and other depressants.

☐ **3.** Use saliva substitutes or sugarless candy or gum to relieve dry mouth.

☐ **4.** Take the drug on an empty stomach.

☐ **5.** Avoid using over-the-counter (OTC) products, except antihistamines and decongestants, without medical permission.

☐ **6.** Discontinue the medication if adverse reactions are troublesome.

Answer: 1, 2, 3

Rationale: Clomipramine, a tricyclic antidepressant used to treat obsessive-compulsive disorder, may cause adverse CNS effects. Therefore, the nurse should warn the client to avoid hazardous activities that require alertness or good coordination until its effects are known. The client should also be instructed to avoid alcohol and other depressants. Dry mouth, a common adverse effect of this medication, can be relieved with saliva substitutes or sugarless candy or gum. The nurse should tell the client to take the medication with meals (not on an empty stomach), especially during the adjustment period, to minimize adverse GI effects. Later, the entire daily dose can be taken at bedtime. The client should check with the physician before taking OTC products because interactions may occur. The nurse should encourage the client to continue therapy, even if adverse reactions are troublesome. The client shouldn't stop taking the medication without medical permission.

Nursing process step: Implementation

Client needs category: Physiological integrity

Client needs subcategory: Pharmacological therapies

Cognitive level: Application

4. A registered nurse caring for a client with generalized anxiety disorder identifies a nursing diagnosis of *Anxiety*. The short-term goal identified is: "The client will identify his physical, emotional, and behavioral responses to anxiety." Which nursing interventions will help the client achieve this goal? Select all that apply.

☐ **1.** Avoid talking about the client's sources of stress.

☐ **2.** Advise the client that consuming one glass of red wine per day may lessen his anxiety.

☐ **3.** Explain to the client that expressing his feelings through journal writing may increase his anxiety.

☐ **4.** Observe the client for overt signs of anxiety.

☐ **5.** Help the client connect anxiety with uncomfortable physical, emotional, or behavioral responses.

☐ **6.** Introduce the client to new strategies for coping with anxiety, such as relaxation techniques and exercise.

Answer: 4, 5, 6

Rationale: The nurse should observe the client for overt signs of anxiety to assess anxiety and establish care priorities. She should also help the client connect anxiety with uncomfortable physical, emotional, or behavioral responses. To modify the automatic response to stress, the client needs to connect the anxiety experience with the unpleasant symptoms. The nurse should also introduce the client to new coping strategies, such as relaxation techniques and exercise, which can enable him to take personal responsibility for making changes. The nurse should work with the client to identify sources of stress—not avoid talking about it. The nurse should advise the client to avoid using caffeine, nicotine, and alcohol to cope with anxiety. Nicotine and caffeine are stimulants; alcohol acts as a depressant but, over time, requires increased use to achieve the desired effect, which may lead to alcohol abuse. The nurse should encourage the client to use a journal to record feelings, behaviors, stressful events, and coping strategies used to address anxiety. Documentation may help the client become aware of his anxiety and the ways in which it affects his overall functioning.

Nursing process step: Implementation

Client needs category: Psychosocial integrity

Client needs subcategory: None

Cognitive level: Application

---

5. A nurse is reviewing information with a client on physical signs and symptoms that may be experienced during a panic attack. Which signs and symptoms should the nurse include? Select all that apply.

☐ **1.** Bradycardia

☐ **2.** Shortness of breath

☐ **3.** Delayed speech

☐ **4.** Dizziness

☐ **5.** Sweating

☐ **6.** GI distress

Answer: 2, 4, 5, 6

Rationale: Panic attacks can produce physical and cognitive symptoms. Such symptoms include a rapid heart beat, shortness of breath or rapid breathing, rapid speech, dizziness or light-headedness, sweating, abdominal pain, nausea, heartburn, and diarrhea (GI distress).

Nursing process step: Implementation

Client needs category: Physiological integrity

Client needs subcategory: Physiological adaptation

Cognitive level: Application

6. A client with a panic disorder is prescribed a monoamine oxidase inhibitor. While reviewing discharge teaching, which dietary restrictions related to this medication would the nurse discuss with the client? Select all that apply.

☐ **1.** Caffeine

☐ **2.** Asparagus

☐ **3.** Sour cream

☐ **4.** Bananas

☐ **5.** Chocolate

☐ **6.** Liver

Answer: 1, 3, 4, 5, 6

Rationale: Foods and beverages containing tyramine, caffeine, and tryptophan must be avoided. Foods that contain such substances include aged cheeses, sour cream, beer, raisins, bananas, pickled or smoked fish, chocolate, and meats (such as liver, sausage, and bologna).

Nursing process step: Implementation

Client needs category: Physiological integrity

Client needs subcategory: Pharmacological therapies

Cognitive level: Application

Mood, adjustment, and dementia disorders

1. A nurse is caring for a client who talks freely about feeling depressed. During an interaction, the nurse hears the client state, "Things will never change." What other indications of hopelessness would the nurse look for? Select all that apply.

☐ **1.** Bouts of anger

☐ **2.** Periods of irritability

☐ **3.** Preoccupation with delusions

☐ **4.** Feelings of worthlessness

☐ **5.** Intense interpersonal relationships

Answer: 1, 2, 4

Rationale: Clients who are depressed and express hopelessness also tend to manifest inappropriate expressions of anger, periods of irritability, and feelings of worthlessness. Preoccupation with delusions is usually seen in clients with schizophrenia; it doesn't typically occur in those who express hopelessness. Intense personal relationships are usually characteristic of clients with borderline personality disorder.

Nursing process step: Data collection

Client needs category: Psychosocial integrity

Client needs subcategory: None

Cognitive level: Analysis

---

2. A nurse interviews the family of a client who's hospitalized with severe depression and suicidal ideation. Which family assessment information is essential to formulating an effective care plan? Select all that apply.

☐ **1.** Physical pain

☐ **2.** Personal responsibilities

☐ **3.** Employment skills

☐ **4.** Communication patterns

☐ **5.** Role expectations

☐ **6.** Current family stressors

Answer: 4, 5, 6

Rationale: When working with the family of a depressed client, it's helpful for the nurse to be aware of the family's communication style, the role expectations for its members, and current family stressors. This information can help to identify family difficulties and teaching points that could benefit the client and the family. Information concerning physical pain, personal responsibilities, and employment skills wouldn't be helpful because these areas aren't directly related to their experience of having a depressed family member.

Nursing process step: Planning

Client needs category: Psychosocial integrity

Client needs subcategory: None

Cognitive level: Analysis

---

3. A client is prescribed sertraline (Zoloft), a selective serotonin reuptake inhibitor. Which information about this drug's adverse effects would the nurse expect when reviewing a medication teaching plan? Select all that apply.

☐ **1.** Agitation

☐ **2.** Agranulocytosis

☐ **3.** Sleep disturbance

☐ **4.** Intermittent tachycardia

☐ **5.** Dry mouth

☐ **6.** Seizures

Answer: 1, 3, 5

Rationale: Common adverse effects of Zoloft include agitation, sleep disturbance, and dry mouth. Agranulocytosis, intermittent tachycardia, and seizures are adverse effects of clozapine (Clozaril).

Nursing process step: Planning

Client needs category: Physiological integrity

Client needs subcategory: Pharmacological therapies

Cognitive level: Comprehension

4. A nurse is observing a client to determine whether he's suffering from dementia or depression. Which information helps the nurse to differentiate between the two? Select all that apply.

☐ **1.** The progression of symptoms is slow.

☐ **2.** The client answers questions with, "I don't know."

☐ **3.** The client acts apathetic and pessimistic.

☐ **4.** The family can't identify when the symptoms first appeared.

☐ **5.** The client's basic personality has changed.

☐ **6.** The client has great difficulty paying attention to others.

Answer: 1, 4, 5, 6

Rationale: Common characteristics of dementia include a slow onset of symptoms, difficulty identifying when the symptoms first occurred, noticeable changes in the client's personality, and impaired ability to pay attention to other people. Apathy, pessimism, and a characteristic response of "I don't know" are symptoms of depression, not dementia.

Nursing process step: Data collection

Client needs category: Psychosocial integrity

Client needs subcategory: None

Cognitive level: Analysis

5. A client has been diagnosed with an adjustment disorder of mixed anxiety and depression. Which nursing diagnoses are associated with a client who has an adjustment disorder? Select all that apply.

☐ **1.** *Activity intolerance*

☐ **2.** *Impaired social interaction*

☐ **3.** *Self-esteem disturbance*

☐ **4.** *Personal identity disturbance*

☐ **5.** *Acute confusion*

☐ **6.** *Impaired memory*

Answer: 2, 3

Rationale: A client with an adjustment disorder is likely to have impaired social interaction and self-esteem disturbance. The other nursing diagnoses aren't related to the diagnosis of adjustment disorder.

Nursing process step: Data collection

Client needs category: Psychosocial integrity

Client needs subcategory: None

Cognitive level: Analysis

6. A physician prescribes lithium for a client diagnosed with bipolar disorder. The nurse needs to provide appropriate education for the client on this drug. Which topics should the nurse cover? Select all that apply.

☐ **1.** The potential for addiction

☐ **2.** Signs and symptoms of drug toxicity

☐ **3.** The potential for tardive dyskinesia

☐ **4.** A low-tyramine diet

☐ **5.** The need to consistently monitor blood levels

☐ **6.** Changes in his mood that may take 7 to 21 days

Answer: 2, 5, 6

Rationale: Client education should cover the signs and symptoms of drug toxicity as well as the need to report them to the physician. The client should be instructed to monitor his lithium levels on a regular basis to avoid toxicity. The nurse should explain that 7 to 21 days may pass before the client notes a change in his mood. Lithium does not have addictive properties. Tyramine is a potential concern to clients taking monoamine-oxidase inhibitors.

Nursing process step: Planning

Client needs category: Physiological integrity

Client needs subcategory: Pharmacological therapies

Cognitive level: Application

Psychotic disorders

1. A nurse is monitoring a client who appears to be hallucinating. Paranoid content is noted in the client's speech and agitated behavior. The client is gesturing at a figure on the television. Which nursing interventions are appropriate? Select all that apply.

☐ **1.** In a firm voice, instruct the client to stop the behavior.

☐ **2.** Reinforce that the client is not in any danger.

☐ **3.** Acknowledge the presence of the hallucinations.

☐ **4.** Instruct other team members to ignore the client's behavior.

☐ **5.** Immediately implement physical restraint procedures.

☐ **6.** Use a calm voice and simple commands.

Answer: 2, 3, 6

Rationale: Using a calm voice, the nurse should reassure the client that he is safe. She shouldn't challenge the client; rather, she should acknowledge his hallucinatory experience. It isn't appropriate to request that the client stop the behavior. Implementing restraints is not warranted at this time. Although the client is agitated, no evidence exists that the client is at risk for harming himself or others.

Nursing process step: Implementation

Client needs category: Psychosocial integrity

Client needs subcategory: None

Cognitive level: Application

2. A client with schizophrenia is taking the atypical antipsychotic medication clozapine (Clozaril). Which signs and symptoms indicate the presence of adverse effects associated with this medication? Select all that apply.

☐ **1.** Sore throat

☐ **2.** Pill-rolling movements

☐ **3.** Polyuria

☐ **4.** Fever

☐ **5.** Polydipsia

☐ **6.** Orthostatic hypotension

Answer: 1, 4

Rationale: Sore throat, fever, and sudden onset of other flulike symptoms are signs of agranulocytosis. The condition is caused by a lack of a sufficient number of granulocytes (a type of white blood cell), which causes the individual to be susceptible to infection. The client's white blood cell count should be monitored at least weekly throughout the course of treatment. Pill-rolling movements can occur in those experiencing extrapyramidal adverse effects associated with antipsychotic medication that has been prescribed for much longer than a medication such as clozapine. Polydipsia (excessive thirst) and polyuria (increased urine) are common adverse effects of lithium. Orthostatic hypotension is an adverse effect of tricyclic antidepressants.

Nursing process step: Data collection

Client needs category: Physiological integrity

Client needs subcategory: Pharmacological therapies

Cognitive level: Application

---

3. A delusional client approaches a nurse, stating, "I am the Easter bunny," and insisting that the nurse refer to him as such. The belief appears to be fixed and unchanging. Which nursing interventions should the nurse implement when working with this client? Select all that apply.

☐ **1.** Consistently use the client's name in interaction.

☐ **2.** Smile at the humor of the situation.

☐ **3.** Agree that the client is the Easter bunny.

☐ **4.** Logically point out why the client could not be the Easter bunny.

☐ **5.** Provide an as-needed medication.

☐ **6.** Provide the client with structured activities.

Answer: 1, 6

Rationale: Continued reality-based orientation is necessary, so it's appropriate to use the client's name in any interaction. Structured activities can help the client refocus and resolve his delusion. The nurse shouldn't contribute to the delusion by going along with the situation or smiling at the humor of the circumstances. Logical arguments and an as-needed medication aren't likely to change the client's beliefs.

Nursing process step: Implementation

Client needs category: Psychosocial integrity

Client needs subcategory: None

Cognitive level: Analysis

4. A physician starts a client on the antipsychotic medication haloperidol (Haldol). The nurse is aware that this medication has extrapyramidal adverse effects. Which measures should the nurse take during Haldol administration? Select all that apply.

- ☐ **1.** Review subcutaneous injection technique.
- ☐ **2.** Closely monitor vital signs, especially temperature.
- ☐ **3.** Observe for increased pacing and restlessness.
- ☐ **4.** Monitor blood glucose levels.
- ☐ **5.** Provide the client with hard candy.
- ☐ **6.** Monitor for signs and symptoms of urticaria.

Answer: 2, 3, 5

Rationale: Neuroleptic malignant syndrome is a life-threatening extrapyramidal adverse effect of antipsychotic medications such as Haldol. It's associated with a rapid increase in temperature. The most common extrapyramidal adverse effect, akathisia, is a form of psychomotor restlessness that can often be seen as pacing. Haldol and the anticholinergic medications that are provided to alleviate its extrapyramidal effects can result in dry mouth. Providing the client with hard candy to suck on can help alleviate this problem. Haldol isn't given subcutaneously and doesn't affect blood glucose levels. Urticaria is not usually associated with Haldol administration.

Nursing process step: Implementation

Client needs category: Physiological integrity

Client needs subcategory: Pharmacological therapies

Cognitive level: Analysis

---

5. A nurse is aware that a client with schizophrenia often progresses through three distinct phases. Place the three phases in ascending chronological order.

| **1.** Active phase |
| **2.** Prodromal phase |
| **3.** Residual phase |

| |
| |
| |

Answer:

| 2. Prodromal phase |
| 1. Active phase |
| 3. Residual phase |

Rationale: Schizophrenia usually progresses through three phases—prodromal, active, and residual. During the prodromal phase, the client exhibits a decline in level of functioning. The active phase involves worsening of the deficits, and the residual phase leads to a return to prodromal phase symptoms, with a blunted affect and impaired role functioning.

Nursing process step: Data collection

Client needs category: Psychosocial integrity

Client needs subcategory: None

Cognitive level: Application

6. While providing a community class on schizophrenia, a nurse reviews factors that increase the client's chances for a positive prognosis. Select all that apply.

☐ **1.** Male gender

☐ **2.** Early onset (in the teen years)

☐ **3.** Sudden disease onset

☐ **4.** Minimal cognitive impairment

☐ **5.** Paranoid schizophrenia subtype

☐ **6.** Good pre-illness functioning

Answer: 3, 4, 5, 6

Rationale: Besides treatment compliance, other factors that portend a good prognosis include female gender, a late or sudden disease onset, minimal cognitive impairment, paranoid schizophrenia subtype, good pre-illness functioning, and a family history of mood disorders (rather than schizophrenia).

Nursing process step: Implementation

Client needs category: Psychosocial integrity

Client needs subcategory: None

Cognitive level: Application

---

7. A nurse is working with a client with schizophrenia who's experiencing auditory hallucinations. Place the interventions in the order that will decrease the client's anxiety. Use all the options.

1. The nurse asks, "What are you experiencing right now?"

2. The nurse encourages the client to tell her when he began hearing voices.

3. The nurse asks the client for permission to discuss the hallucinations.

4. The nurse asks the client if he has taken drugs or alcohol recently.

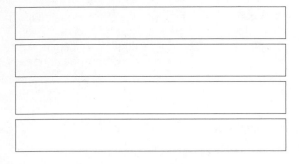

Answer:

3. The nurse asks the client for permission to discuss the hallucinations.

1. The nurse asks, "What are you experiencing right now?"

4. The nurse asks the client if he has taken drugs or alcohol recently.

2. The nurse encourages the client to tell her when he began hearing voices.

Rationale: Asking the client for permission to discuss the hallucinations promotes trust, which is an essential first step in communicating with clients who are hallucinating. When the nurse asks what the client is experiencing, the question should be based on the nurse's observation of some cue (such as eyes looking around the room). Relaying this observation to the client will help in understanding the symptoms, further increase trust, and decrease the client's perception that the nurse has extraordinary power to read his mind. Asking the client if he has taken drugs or alcohol recently will help in determining the source of the current experience. Lastly, the client is encouraged to tell the nurse when the voices started. Once trust is established, the client will be more comfortable discussing the past.

Nursing process step: Implementation

Client needs category: Psychosocial integrity

Client needs subcategory: None

Cognitive level: Application

Substance abuse, eating disorders, and impulse control disorders

1. A nurse is assessing a client who has been diagnosed with bulimia nervosa. The nurse is aware that this disorder is characterized by eating binges accompanied by which symptoms? Select all that apply.

☐ **1.** Guilt

☐ **2.** Dental caries

☐ **3.** Self-induced vomiting

☐ **4.** Weight loss

☐ **5.** Normal weight

☐ **6.** Introverted behavior

Answer: 1, 2, 3, 5

Rationale: Guilt, dental caries, self-induced vomiting, and normal weight are all associated with bulimia nervosa. Weight loss and introverted behavior are associated with anorexia nervosa.

Nursing process step: Data collection

Client needs category: Psychosocial integrity

Client needs subcategory: None

Cognitive level: Analysis

---

2. While checking a client upon arrival to the emergency department, a nurse is concerned that the client may be under the influence of amphetamines. Which symptoms may indicate the influence of amphetamines? Select all that apply.

☐ **1.** Depressed affect

☐ **2.** Diaphoresis

☐ **3.** Shallow respirations

☐ **4.** Hypotension

☐ **5.** Tremors

☐ **6.** Dilated pupils

Answer: 2, 3, 5, 6

Rationale: In a client under the influence of amphetamines, data collection findings may include euphoria, diaphoresis, shallow respirations, tremors, dilated pupils, dry mouth, anorexia, tachycardia, hypertension, hyperthermia, seizures, and altered mental status.

Nursing process step: Data collection

Client needs category: Psychosocial integrity

Client needs subcategory: None

Cognitive level: Application

3. A client admitted for the second time this winter with pneumonia has stated, "I'm really ready to kick this habit of smoking but I don't know where to begin." A nurse explains that there are several options to assist a client in smoking cessation. Select all that apply.

☐ **1.** Use of nicotine replacement (nicotine gum, transdermal patches, nasal sprays and inhalers)

☐ **2.** Use of clonidine or diazepam (Valium) to mimic the effects of nicotine

☐ **3.** Use of alcohol to blunt the effect caused by withdrawal from nicotine

☐ **4.** Behavioral therapies and treatments

☐ **5.** Acupuncture

☐ **6.** Identifying coping skills and then seeking exposure to a smoking environment to test these skills

Answer: 1, 2, 4, 5

Rationale: Use of nicotine replacement through patches, gum, sprays, and inhalers may relieve withdrawal symptoms. Nicotine mimicking agents, such as clonidine and diazepam, are successful for many clients. Other clients report success after acupuncture treatment, and behavioral interventions can play a key role in treating nicotine dependency. The treatment with the most success includes a combination of pharmacologic and behavioral therapies. To help prevent relapse, the client should avoid substituting one form of dependency for another and exposure to smoking environments and smokers.

Nursing process step: Implementation

Client needs category: Psychosocial integrity

Client needs subcategory: None

Cognitive level: Application

---

4. Which interventions would be supportive for a client with a nursing diagnosis of *Imbalanced nutrition: Consuming less than the body requires due to dysfunctional eating patterns?* Select all that apply.

☐ **1.** Provide small, frequent feedings.

☐ **2.** Monitor weight fluctuations.

☐ **3.** Allow the client to skip meals until the antidepressant levels are therapeutic.

☐ **4.** Encourage journaling to promote the expression of feelings.

☐ **5.** Monitor the client at mealtimes and for an hour after meals.

☐ **6.** Encourage the client to eat three substantial meals per day.

Answer: 1, 2, 4, 5

Rationale: Smaller meals may be better tolerated by the client and will gradually increase her daily caloric intake. The nurse should monitor the client's weight because an anorexic will hide weight loss. Anorexics are emotionally restrained and afraid of their feelings, so journaling can be a powerful tool that assists in recovery. Anorexic clients are obsessed with gaining weight and will skip all meals if given the opportunity. Because of self-starvation, they seldom can tolerate large meals three times per day.

Nursing process step: Implementation

Client needs category: Psychosocial integrity

Client needs subcategory: None

Cognitive level: Analysis

5. While collecting data on a client who was diagnosed with impulse control disorder (and who displays violent, aggressive, and assaultive behavior), the nurse can expect to find which data? Select all that apply.

☐ **1.** The client functions well in other areas of his life.

☐ **2.** The degree of aggressiveness is out of proportion to the stressor.

☐ **3.** The client often uses a stressor to justify the violent behavior.

☐ **4.** The client has a history of parental alcoholism and a chaotic, abusive family life.

☐ **5.** The client shows no remorse about his inability to control his behavior.

Rationale: A client with an impulse control disorder who displays violent, aggressive, and assaultive behavior generally functions well in other areas of his life. The degree of the client's aggressiveness is disproportionate to the stressor, and the client commonly has a history of parental alcoholism, as well as a chaotic family life. The client often verbalizes sincere guilt and remorse for the aggressive behavior.

Nursing process step: Data collection

Client needs category: Psychosocial integrity

Client needs subcategory: None

Cognitive level: Application